FEEL GOOD HEALTH

FEEL GOOD HEALTH

THE BODY & MIND GUIDE
FOR LIVING HEALTHY ALL YEAR

DOMINIC GAZIANO, M.D.

Copyright © 2007 Feel Good Health Group

While a great deal of care has beeen taken to provide accurate and current information, the ideas, suggestions, general principals and conclusions presented in this text are subject to local, state and federal laws and regulations, court cases and any revisions of same. The reader should consult medical council regarding any points of health – this publication should not be used as a substitute for individual health advice from the reader's health care provider.

Publisher: Dominic Gaziano, M.D
Executive Editor: Melissa Giovagnoli
Managing Editor: Brenna Walters
Associate Editor: Derrick Sorles
Cover & Interior Design: Kerry LaCoste, LaCosteDesign.com
Photography: iStockphoto®

Published by Feel Good Health Group

All rights reserved. The text of this publication, or any part thereof, may not be reproduced in any manner whatsoever without written permission from the publisher.

Printed in the United States of America

Library of Congress Cataloging-in-Publication Data

Dominic Gaziano, M.D.
www.feelgoodhealthnow.com
Feel Good Health: the body & mind guide for living healthy all year/Dominic Gaziano, M.D.
    p. cm.
    Includes bibliographical references and index.

Print ISBN-13: 978-1-948543-72-9
Digital ISBN-13: 978-1-948543-73-6

THIS BOOK IS DEDICATED

TO MY PARENTS WHO INSTILLED IN ME
AN EMOTIONAL STABILITY THAT HELPED ME
GET THROUGH THE RIGORS OF MEDICAL
TRAINING AND LIFE;

AND TO MY BROTHERS PHIL, MIKE,
TODD, AND TOM WHO HELPED INSPIRE
IN ME A PASSION FOR SCIENCE,
NATURE AND SPORT.

FEEL GOOD
HEALTH
CONTENTS

7
WELCOME TO FEEL GOOD HEALTH

11
HOW TO USE THIS BOOK

15
FEEL GOOD SUMMER

45
FEEL GOOD FALL

81
FEEL GOOD WINTER

117
FEEL GOOD SPRING

149
HEALTH & HAPPINESS PLANNER

154
INDEX

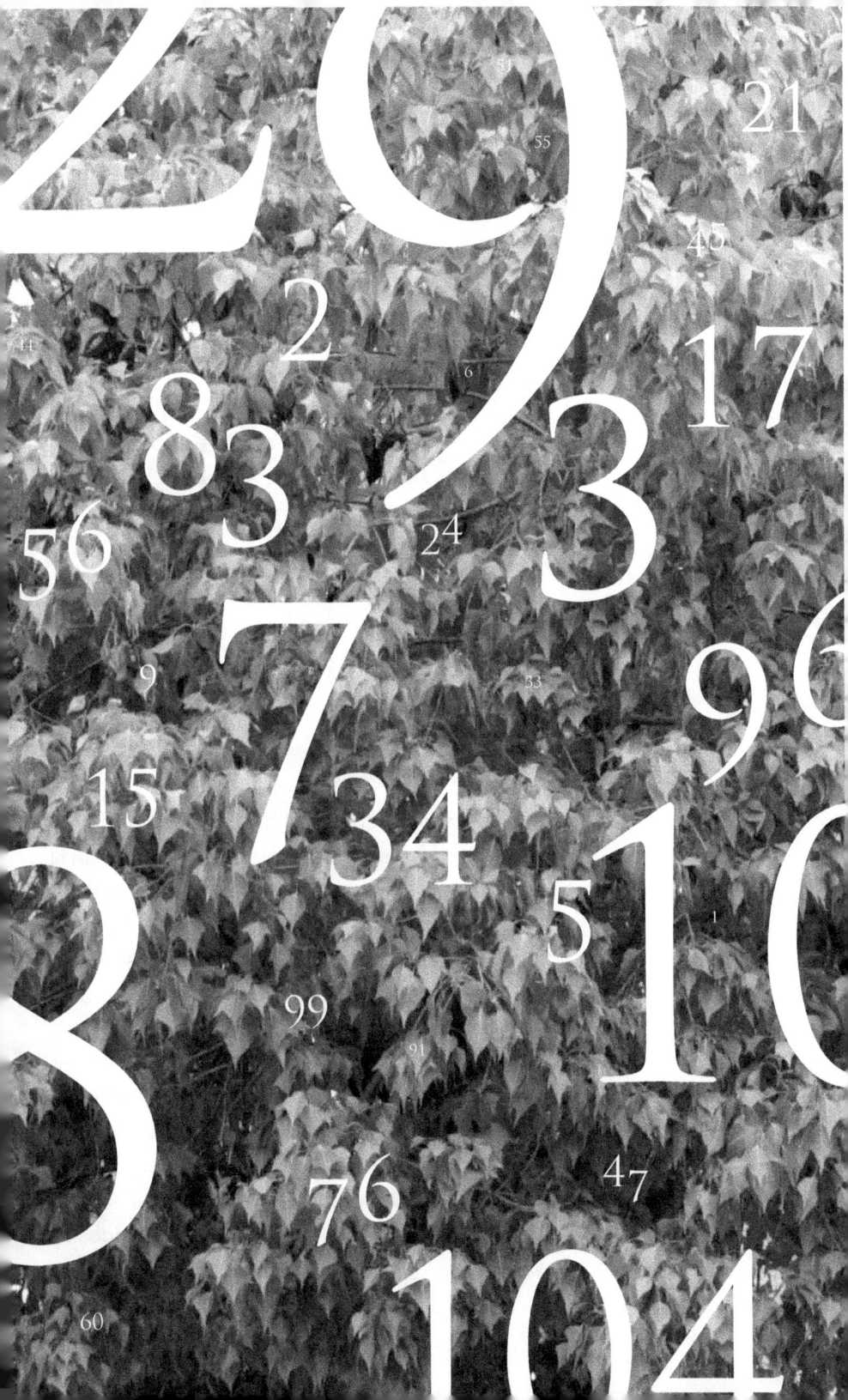

WELCOME TO FEEL GOOD HEALTH

In our modern world, technology and wealth have made us more sedentary and overweight. We have nearly eradicated polio, small pox, and tuberculoses, yet we have a raging epidemic of obesity. Additionally, our nutrition is poor and a world diabetic epidemic, both in children and adults, is predicted to continue to rise as well.

While modern technology allows us to check email from anywhere in the world, receive phone calls at any time, and fly miles away for a meeting and still be home the same night, the stress of keeping up in a fast-paced society has taken its toll on both our bodies and minds. Our lives today are so over booked that we skip workouts, eat fat and cholesterol laden convenience foods, and do not listen when our bodies are telling us to stop. Our unhealthy habits have left us depressed, overwhelmed and overweight. It doesn't have to be this way.

As an internal medicine specialist, I have seen the end results of unhealthy habits first hand. I treat patients with heart conditions, strokes, lung cancer and a host of other illnesses that could have been prevented with proper nutrition and a little more activity. After listening to my patients complain that they don't have time to work out or prepare healthy meals, I knew that there was a way to introduce better eating habits, activity, and fun to my patients' lives. Feel Good Health is my answer to people who have a hard time eating right and exercising. It is a tool and a guide to living better.

Many of my patients want to do the right thing, but they hear conflicting information from television reports or on the Internet, and they do not know where to turn. A few decades ago it was no fat and carbs were good, then it was low calorie, then suddenly carbs became the biggest weight loss enemy, then food combination was in, and then volumetric and on and on. Faced will all these choices people should be able to turn to their doctor for advice, but doctors' visits only last an average of seven minutes. This book speaks to the need that my patients have voiced about how to lead a healthy lifestyle with their hectic schedules.

So what is Feel Good Health and how does it work? It's a simple way to develop a healthy lifestyle that makes you feel good on the inside and out.

It's based on the concept that getting healthy should not be such an arduous task. You do not have to feel deprived or dedicate all your time to preparing tasteless meals. In fact, getting healthy can be easy and fun. I wrote this book to illustrate just that; living healthy is simple, fun and makes you feel great!

This is different from other books out there that provide knowledge about medical systems or books that provide diet guides. Feel Good Health guides you through each season, providing goals,

WELCOME TO FEEL GOOD HEALTH

inspiration for achieving those goals, and bi-weekly tips. The tips are your step-by-step guide to achieving and maintaining a healthy lifestyle, mentally and physically.

The tips address your mental and physical health while reminding you to have fun throughout each season. To get the most of this book I ask you to choose two tips a week to gradually incorporate into your new healthy lifestyle. This way you will be able to more powerfully sustain a new way of living a healthy life without a lot of effort.

I encourage you to try these tips with your family and friends, creating a Feel Good Health community. I also give you the tools to build a healthier network of co-workers, friends, neighbors, local merchants and medical professionals to turn to for informational and emotional support.

The mission of this book is to provide you with the information and strategies to help you achieve a healthier life in body and mind. I will provide you with tools to be successful, more youthful and have more energy.

This body and mind guide will elevate your health knowledge and show you how to implement habits that improve your overall health. It will help you achieve a healthy state of mind and body through daily fitness and nutrition habits and by implementing preventative techniques.

Is it going to be hard to master these health concepts? Don't worry, the fact that you picked up this book means you are half way there. You have probably already been exposed too much of this information. We have just organized the information and presented it in a fun way that makes the concept of healthy living a snap. These principles are not like trying to understand the area in an isosceles triangle. Living a healthy lifestyle is not as hard as you think. It can actually be fun.

In the course of reading this book, your overall health will improve as you implement these healthy practices for the rest of your life.

Each season, I will give tips to improve your mental health, nutrition knowledge, fitness level, and expand your understanding of preventative health management. To achieve these goals, I will provide you with two tips per week throughout the season. You get to choose when and how to use each tip. Incorporating these tips into your life style will slowly remove roadblocks to achieving better health. I will help you set a reasonable timetable to realize these goals. This is not a radical diet that forces you to completely change over night. This book will teach you to give up bad habits, replacing them with new healthy habits over time.

I have used my years of experience in medicine and my passion for health in writing this book. Additionally, research for this book was provided by the best sources, including the American Dietary Association, peer-reviewed journals, American Heart Association, and the American Cancer Society.

HOW TO USE THIS BOOK

It is advised to skim through the whole book first for an overall understanding. Once you have an understanding, I recommend reading the appropriate season and getting to work with the tips. Twenty-six lifestyle tips have been provided for each season. At the end of each season, I have included a schedule for you to fill-out with tips. You should incorporate two tips a week into your schedule. Remember this is supposed to be fun, so be flexible with yourself but try to stick to your schedule as much as you can.

Each tip will fit into the general category of mind, body, or fun. The mind tips help you achieve a peaceful, productive state of mind and help you manage stress. The body tips help to achieve a healthy body through nutrition, fitness and preventative medicine implementation. The fun tips can be sprinkled throughout the season to make sure you are enjoying yourself and inspire you to be healthy.

These fun tips are also intended to remind you to connect with your community and keep laughing as you transition into your new healthy lifestyle. Some of the tips may appear to overlap, incorporating benefits for your mind and body – even better. Don't get caught up in what category each tip fits in, just make sure you do two tips each week.

When deciding which tips to do and in what order, pick your vacation week first and at least one weekend getaway for each season, even if you don't go away physically. You can put the fun tips in the vacation week.

As you incorporate the tips make sure that you understand the tip and know how to incorporate it into your life. If you want to modify any tip, please feel free to make the tips work for you, but try to stick to the basic premises. If you do modify the tip, I would love to know how you did with it. I welcome your feedback or suggestions. Feel free to visit my blog at www.feelgoodhealthnow.com often for many additional and helpful health aides.

If you miss a week, don't worry, but try to catch up the next week. Read the tips and try to understand them so you can use the tips for the rest of you life. Then, do your best to incorporate your new habits in to your live. You control how you integrate the tips for each season and how you live your healthy lifestyle.

It is said that success in anything is 1% inspiration and 99% perspiration so we need some inspiration along the way, which is why I have provided fun tips in each season.

We will also inspire, motivate and hopefully get you through those tough times and crises. We want to make you stronger mentally with stress management strategies and by showing you how to build the right support team.

HOW TO USE THIS BOOK

This book is a journey of incorporating healthy habits. When you have finished reading this book and have practiced the tips, commit them to memory so that they are available for life. Your health understanding and healthy lifestyle skills will only improve from this moment. Good luck and Feel Good reading.

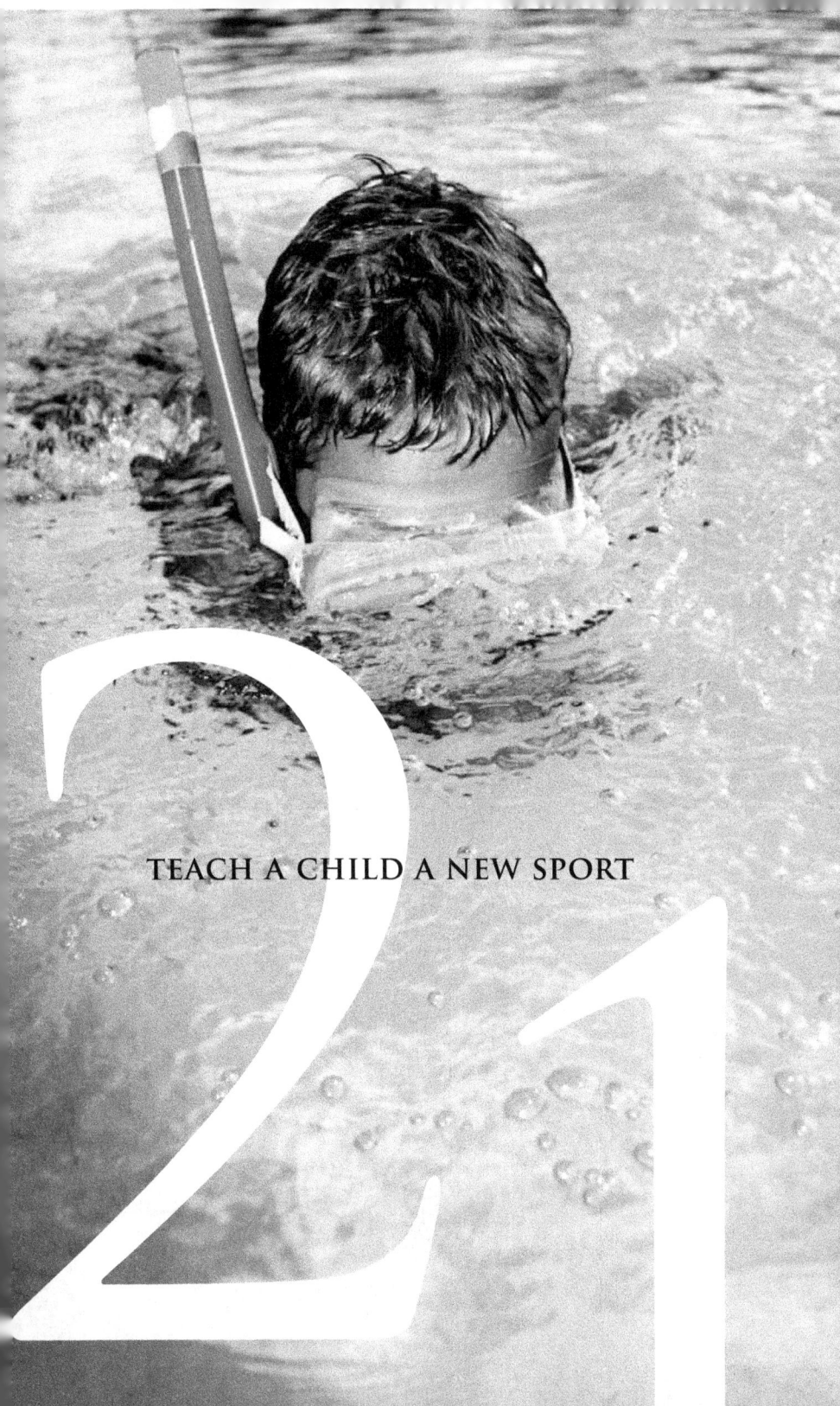

21
TEACH A CHILD A NEW SPORT

FEEL GOOD SUMMER

SUMMER

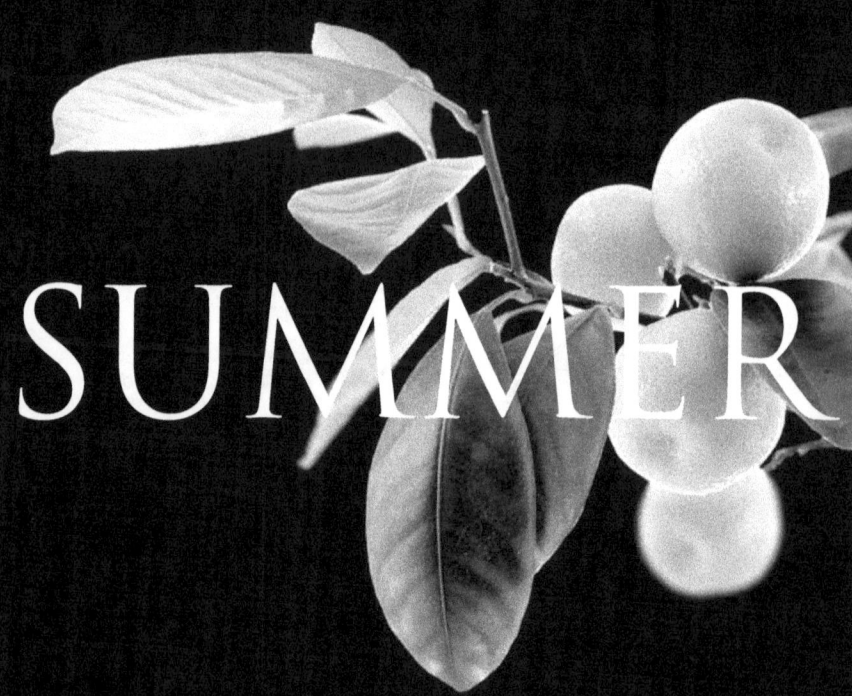

'Recreate the pure passion, fun and adventure
of youthful summers to keep you healthy and happy'

– *Dominic Gaziano, M.D.*

GOALS FOR SUMMER

That's What Friends Are For:
Increase the strength of interpersonal supports (friends, family, and co-workers) by hosting cookouts and learning to use nature and the outdoors to relieve stress and to help you to relax.

**Did You Really Think
"All You Can Eat Bacon" Was the Right Idea:**
Determine your ideal weight and develop a
weight management lifestyle by incorporating fresh foods and switching to healthier options.

It's Go Time:
Expand your fitness community by inviting
friends, co-workers, and family to join you in trying new sports, increasing your daily activity.

Sun, Bugs, and Allergens, Oh My:
Learn how to protect yourself from the dangers
of summertime fun.

FEEL GOOD SUMMER

Summer is finally here. The memories come flooding back. Take a minute. When was your best summer of the past? Was it last summer? Was it when you were seven or fifteen or perhaps twenty-one? Were you away from your parents at summer camp? Did you travel to some warm beach with your family? Did you BBQ and host block parties or did you meet that special someone and steal a kiss in the woods or spend warm nights strolling on the beach?

My best summer was when I was 20, home from college and relieved, briefly, from the rigors of my pre-medical studies. I was a lifeguard at Berry Hills Country club and life was good. I swam every morning and even had free access to the country club golf course on the Montanans of West Virginia. The kitchen chef would make a special chicken dish for me every day and I thought life couldn't get much better. That summer I got a hole-in-one on the golf course and even had a special summer fling.

What does that have to do with health? Everything. You need to have fun to stay healthy! If you are happy and enjoying life, you are more inclined to take care of yourself and maintain your healthy habits.

Close your eyes remember your best summer. Now, open your eyes. Let's help you relive that memory.

Summer is a time to venture out and explore. The tips this season will help you explore a more vibrant, healthy and fun way of living. Focus on exploring with your friends and by yourself. Use whatever nature is around you to help relieve the stress in your life. If you live in the country then nature is all around you. You city dwellers can go to the parks, lakes, beaches, and recreational areas. I recommend getting done with work a little early one day and walking in the park alone or with a friend for a moment of peace.

Take in sunsets, do meditation, and become more infused with the rhythms of nature. Try to skip the TV on these days. Truly enjoy and appreciate nature. Get to know your neighborhood by finding a walking or running path. Talk to the fruit and vegetable expert at the neighborhood grocery store or at the farmers market. Summer is a great time to incorporate fresh foods into your diet and increase the visual appeal of your meals by choosing a variety of colorful fruits and vegetables.

With block parties, festivals, and backyard BBQs, summer is also a time to connect with people. Use this time to solidify support relationships with friends and family. Do something really nice for them when it is easier to do things outside in the warm summer air. You need friends year round, so take time to do something nice for them when you can.

TIPS FROM THE M.D.

Severe Allergic Reactions

Since we spend more time outside in the summer, we are exposed to more insects, like bees and wasps that can sting us. We are also exposed to outdoor allergens. If you are prone to allergies, you should take steps to prevent or treat possible allergic reactions. If you are allergic to bee stings and you have been told you have severe anaphylactic reactions, it is best to have your doctor prescribe you an Ana kit.

An anaphylactic reaction is a severe allergic reaction to an allergen, or something we are allergic to. The symptoms include fever, rash, difficulty breathing, and chest pain. If the heart is affected, the blood pressure could drop quickly, and you will need to seek immediate medical attention; this is a medical emergency. An Ana kit is an injection of epinephrine to counteract the life threatening reaction.

You can administer this injection yourself if you get a severe allergic reaction. Having this on hand can save your life. If you have been prescribed an Ana kit in the past, make sure you know where it is and it has not expired.

Recipe for your Summer of Exploration Cocktail

Ingredients
 1 part Relaxed Attitude
 3 parts Outdoor Activities
 3 parts Summer Fresh Foods
 2 parts Fun Time With Friends and Family

Directions
Mix outdoor activities together with summer fresh foods, blend fun time with family and friends together with a relaxed attitude. Garnish with a cocktail umbrella. Best served with friends.

Summertime Inspirations
Don't forget to find inspiration to get into the summer mood. I recommend a few movies to help recreate that carefree time of summer. "Endless Summer" and "A Separate Peace" are a couple of classics and my personal favorites.

Summer is a time to get out your summer reading list and try to spend time quietly reading and relaxing. On top of my summer reading list is To Kill a Mocking Bird. It is infused with small town country summer images. These images stay with me all year long and get me through the colder winter months. It is important to embrace and build that invincible summer in body and mind and store it up for the winter.

Great Summers of the Past:
Now for some great summers of the past — there have been many major accomplishments during the summer. The most memorable of which are the summer of 1985 when music legends got together

to host a concert that raised $100 million for the victims of famine in Ethiopia.

Not many people can forget where they were in the summer of 1969 when we first landed on the moon. On July 20, 1969, America squinted up at the heavens, trying to see an extra speck on the moon. This was truly uplifting. If NASA could roll up their sleeves and bear the heat of the summer to put a man on the moon, you can conquer the uncharted territory of your new jogging path.

What could symbolize summer more than the tropical paradise of Hawaii, which was added as a state in, you guessed it, the summer of 1959 on August 21.

With all these great summers behind us it is time to look forward to this summer. This is the summer of you. It is the time for you to adopt a fun and healthy life style. Outlined below are the goals for the summer and the tips to help you get here. This is the summer of healthy exploration. Enjoy it!

TIPS FROM THE M.D.

Contact Dermatitis

You should avoid plants with three leaves clusters, which are growing on trees or on vines. This could be poison ivy. A poison ivy rash is an eruptive rash. To prevent contact dermatitis (an infected skin rash) or to at least limit its spread, wash the areas of contact vigorously with soap and water. Over the counter treatments are available at a pharmacy. Make sure you how to recognize the poison ivy plant, because avoiding it altogether is much easier than treating a rash.

FRESH PICKED SUMMER TIPS

1. Eat Fresh Berries To Increase Your Antioxidant Levels

Almost all berries have a high level of antioxidants. Heading up this list is the blueberry, a fantastic summer berry that stays in season all summer long. Eat blueberries fresh and sprinkle them on your cereal in the morning or use blueberries to make healthy blueberry shakes.

Berries have powerful anti-aging properties, including antioxidants. Want to feel great and look younger, cozy up with some blackberries, strawberries, raspberries, or cherries. Berries can be found just about any where in the summer. Make berry salads with any of these or find recipes that incorporate berries.

Not a berry fan? Antioxidants also come in the following tasty packages: broccoli, tomatoes, red grapes, spinach, tea, carrots, soy and whole grains.

TIPS FROM THE M.D.

What Are Antioxidants?

Just what are antioxidants and how can they help prevent aging and the artery-clogging process known as atherosclerosis?

Antioxidants are disease-fighting compounds that prevent free radicals from causing more damage. Free radicals are unstable molecules that cause cellular damage because they wiz around a cell slamming into other compounds and stealing electrons, rendering these compounds unstable. The compound then tries to gain stability by stealing someone else's electron, which leads to a domino effect across the cell. In the cellular world, instability is a bad thing.

Free radicals occur as a normal part of cell function, but are also introduced at higher levels from outside influences such as foods high in saturated fats, simple sugars, and smoking. Antioxidants stabilize free radicals by donating their own electrons, thus preventing massive electron stealing from another cell.

Antioxidants can decrease the risk of age related neurological conditions, lower blood pressure, help the immune system to be stronger, and can help prevent many types of cancer through the prevention of DNA damage.

2. Talk To the Produce Expert at the Fruit and Vegetable Stand

Ask how they choose their produce. Find out where the fruits and vegetables come from. Have them guide you through how to choose the best fruits and vegetables. From touch and sight, to smell, there are different ways to tell when a fruit or vegetable is at its peak.

The American Dietary association states that the fruit you choose can be fresh, canned, frozen or dried, but in the summer take advantage of all the fresh fruit available. Talk to your grocer and get to know them by name. Ask for him when you go to the grocery store and learn what produce they recommend for that week.

How many fruits and vegetables do you need in a day? Well, you need about five to nine servings of fruits and vegetables a day. Visit My Pyramid at Mypyramid.gov to receive specific information that pertains to you individually.

3. Take a Thirty-Minute Walk In a New Neighborhood

Exploring new neighborhoods allows you to experience someone else's world without having to travel very far. Maybe your friend lives in another neighborhood and they can show you their favorite walking paths or trails. Be adventurous, but safe. Walk during the day in safe neighborhoods and if you don't know the area, carry your cell phone with you and notify a friend of where you will be. Breaking your normal routine and walking in another environment will clear your head and give you a new perspective. Strolling is great, but try a brisk walk to get that heart rate up.

4. Eat at an Organic or Raw Healthy Restaurant

I know a raw food restaurant sounds like a hoax, but the raw food movement is gaining popularity. Raw food is never heated above 118 degrees and is unprocessed. You never know, you might love it, or at least get some new ideas. If you are not hot on the raw food idea, try to find an organic or healthy restaurant.

Unfortunately, many restaurants simply heat-up frozen products and serve them to you. I'm not just talking about fast food; these are actual sit down resultants. Their food can be loaded with preservatives and fat. Yuck!

Depending on where you live, these raw or organic restaurants may be difficult to find. If you can't locate one, try to find a restaurant that is committed to and preparing quality healthy meals.

Find restaurants in your area that prepare food fresh everyday. When in doubt, chefs and kitchen managers can be excellent resources and most are happy to tell you about the food they prepare. While you have their ear, ask them what they think is the best and most healthy dish.

5. **Get a Facial To Prepare Your Skin For Summer**

Not only will you look and feel great, but you can also learn how to properly care for your skin all year long. Most skin care professionals are happy to recommend products that will work well with your skin type. Facials are not just about washing your face and slapping on some moisturizer. A good estitition will spend time evaluating your skin and clearing up can clogged pores that you may have. They will also massage your face, hitting those all-important pressure points. You will leave relaxed, rejuvenated, and glowing with radiant new skin.

Gentlemen – you're expected to participate too. Many spas now offer Gentlemen-only treatments. In general, facials help regenerate parched skin and return a natural and healthy glow to skin. Treatment can vary from a Hot Stone facial to an acne relief facial. Special treatment will vary depending on where you live. Be sure to talk to a skin care professional to determine which treatment is right for your skin type.

6. Fitness With Animals

Study after study has shown that animals have a calming effect on us humans (unless you are house breaking). Enjoy outdoor activities with your pup. Take a long walk, go to the dog park or beach, and be social with other dog owners. If you don't have a dog, tag along with a dog owning friend or ask to pet sit for an afternoon. A good game of chase is great aerobic activity. Did you know that there is a place called "lets pet puppies" that lets you socialize a young pup by playing with them.

Ready for a bigger animal and a bigger challenge. Go horseback riding.

If you have ever done any real horseback riding (and I'm not talking about the ponies that circle around), you know what a great workout it can be. Horseback riding not only exercises your body, but your mind as well. Learning how to control your horse and use your body can be a mental and physical challenge. Even with the challenges, being with horses out in nature can be incredibly relaxing.

Scared of dogs or horseback riding? Go to the zoo and watch the orangutans. At least they will make you laugh.

7. Try Methods To Increase Your Intimacy With Your Significant Other

If you presently have a significant other, you may feel the need to strengthen your relationship sexually. Treat the bedroom as a protected environment where you can be honest about what is working sexually. Discuss with your partner what you enjoy most and any problems or issues you are having. If you feel the need, sometimes talking with a therapist can remove stress and help you and your partner communicate better.

8. Spend Time In the Park Sitting Alone

Take a few moments for yourself. The rhythms of nature can give you a lot. Sit still for fifteen minutes without moving. Just breath slowly in and out, following your breath as you inhale and exhale. You can do it. Sit and enjoy the moment. Watch people, animals and enjoy being in nature. Just be with your own thoughts – and stop mentally reviewing your to do list.

Use this time to clear your head and let go of any issues that are not worth stressing about. Time to decompress and be with your own thoughts is so important to your mental heath. Unfortunately, in our busy lives we forget to stop and appreciate a few moments of quiet.

9. Sit In the Park With Someone Special

I know, I just said to sit alone, but trust me, both can be therapeutic. You can sit with anyone: your special someone, your child, your parent or grandparent, or even a friend. Enjoy a still moment in this person's company. Americans lead such a hectic life that we sometimes forget to enjoy the company of friends and family. Sit together with no distractions and really be present with your loved one. Talk about what you see together or take the time to update each other about what's been going on in your lives.

When we make plans with friends and even family members, we forget that there are other things to do together than grab drinks or dine out. Invite a friend to stroll through the park with you and find a comfortable spot just to sit and relax.

10. Have a Skin Physical

It's time to show some skin. You should do a general body survey, looking for dark moles that may have changed in color or gotten bigger lately. If you have been a sun worshiper most of your life, then it is time to take a closer look at your skin.

Many skin conditions heal themselves all on their own. The skin is a pretty remarkable organ, but some times it is necessary to see your primary care doctor. Yes, your regular doctor can help treat a number of skin issues. It's time to see your doctor if a new rash appears or if you notice any changes in your skin. They may refer you to a dermatologist for specific issues such as acne, atopic dermatitis, rosacea, or skin cancers.

11. Find Out Your Ideal Body Weight

There are people walking around that don't even know they are overweight. We have really lost touch with the amount of weight we should be carrying around. It is important to know how much you should weigh for several reasons. Aesthetics aside, your extra weight will negatively affect your health. When you are overweight, you increase your changes of having heart disease and diabetes. You also put unnecessary stress on your back and joints.

To calculate your ideal weight you can use the following as a general rule:

Female Body Mass Index
For the first five feet you should weigh 100lbs. Add five pounds to every inch thereafter.

Male Body Mass Index
For the first 5 feet you should weigh 106lbs. Add six pounds to every inch thereafter.

Are you surprised at what you should weigh? While I don't want you to be obsessed with a number on a scale, it is important to know a starting point. Once you know your weight and your goal weight then you can begin to establish a plan to either get closer to your goal or maintain your healthy weight. Go ahead and take the challenge. See the chart as the end of this section for your ideal weight.

TIPS FROM THE M.D.

Determining If You Can Exercise

Most people are physically able to exercise. However, as we know, most people have some excuse not to exercise. In general, consult with your doctor before you exercise. If you have any chest pain or arm pain - especially left arm or neck pain when you start an exercise regimen, stop exercising and contact your doctor. If you experience any significant shortness of breath, wheezing, chest tightness contact you doctor. If you experience initial bone or joint pains you should consult your doctor.

12. Watch Movies and Videos That Remind You Of Summer Fun To Motivate You To Start Exercising

Whether it is watching "Chariots of Fire" to encourage you to run, or "Step into Liquid" to motivate you to surf, movies are a great way to get inspired. You might want to purchase a new workout video or posting a picture of a thinner you somewhere that will remind you to get up, get active and get you into that summer spirit.

Speaking of summer spirit, when is the last time you watched "Endless Summer"? It has been a summer classic since it was first released in 1966. Since then, several other summer classics have entered the cultural psyche. Most summer movies are upbeat and fun and if they feature music by The Beach Boys, even better. Find your own favorite summer movies and music to get you inspired.

13. Prepare a Romantic Dinner With Candlelight Outside

Take the time to set-up a romantic space for yourself and your significant other. Sit outside on your balcony or patio and enjoy fresh, sensuous foods. Don't have anyone to share this special evening with? - Do it for yourself, sit outside and enjoy your time alone. It is important to pamper yourself.

14. Exercise at Dawn at Your Home or Gym

Oh, the agony of leaving bed before the sun is up. Get over it. You will benefit all day long from a morning work out. Not only will you get that work out out of the way before life creeps up and distracts you, but you will also feel energized throughout your busy day.

Try a morning golf game or run through the park and enjoy the sunrise.

If you already have a great work out schedule in place, then don't fix what is not broken. However consider this, many people report appetite regulation and increased energy when they work out in the morning. There are also reports that suggest our circadian rhythms (our 24-hour biological cycle) are set for morning work outs.

The most important thing is to work out and if you work out in the morning then you can check it off your list and you can save the energy you would have spent making excuses to not work out later.

15. Watch the Different Phases of Sunset

Nothing compares to a summer sunset when everything is bathed in golden light. Watch the sky take on brilliant red and orange colors as the sun says goodnight.

Do you know there is a name for what causes all those colors? Mie Scattering is a formula that calculates the scattering of electromagnetic radiation by spherical particles. These particles transmit at the wavelength that reflects red. It is these little guys that light up the sky with that brilliant red hue. What about sunrise, why is the sunset much more colorful? It's actually the sun's fault. The sun heats up the earth during daylight hours and changes the relative humidity, wind speeds and turbulence which affects the amount of dust, the reflector of all those colors.

Now that you know all of this, research more about the sunset, or rise, but make sure you get out there and enjoy it. With the longer summer days, you will have more time to reach the best viewing spots in your town. Watch along, with friends, or make it a family trip.

16. Go To a Baseball Game

Summer is not complete without a trip to the ball park. Games can be thrilling and invigorating, especially if you are watching a close game. They can also be relaxing as you sit out in the summer sun and experience one of America's favorite pastimes. You don't even need to be a baseball fantastic to enjoy going to a game. Games are very social events. They are a great excuse to get outside on a weekend or take off a little early from work. Take your family or go with friends. Either way, don't miss this seasonal staple – Just limit your intake of hotdog(s), nacho(s), and beer. Remember your sunscreen too.

17. Go Out Dancing Outdoors

Why not? Have fun and make a fool of yourself. If you're up for it take lessons and really impress your friends and family.

There is a reason that the dance revolution is keeping kids fit. Dancing is great exercise and it is fun. It is also a good way to let off steam and de-stress from a rough day a work. Burn calories, laugh and dance your way to happiness. Turn on music that makes you want to move and get into it.

Many cities have outdoor summer dance venues. If you cannot find one, create your own dance group with your friends or turn on your radio and dance around your backyard. Make sure you are having fun and don't hesitate to invite friends and make it a social event.

18. Use Sunscreen Every Day

Do you remember when women used to put olive oil on their skin to tan? You can usually point them out now. Sunscreen should be a no brainer by now. Whether it's cloudy or not, it is imperative for you to use a sunscreen daily. It is the number one thing you can do for yourself to slow down the aging process.

You should always use SPF 15 or above on your face. Apply sunscreen about twenty or thirty minutes before going outside. About one ounce of sunscreen should be used to cover the arms, legs, neck and face of an average adult. Most sunscreen needs to be applied every 2 hours.

Tanning is an appropriate time to fake it. There are several great products out there that give you a natural glow with out damaging your skin or increasing your risk for skin cancers.

19. Take a Healthy Cooking Class

One of the best things you can do is take time to cook with someone you care about. It will increase your communication skills, as well as your "fun factor." There is nothing like learning a new recipe and co-creating a new dish with someone. In only a couple of hours, you will have a healthy meal and lots of memories to share. Check out local stores that offer classes, such as William Sonoma, Chopping Block, Sur La Table, and Caphalon.

Can't find a class? Get a group of friends together and each commit to learn a healthy dish. Take turns teaching each other.

20. Buy a Healthy Cookbook

There are thousands out there. Find a health cookbook that speaks to you. Make it a habit to try one new recipe a month. Invite friends over to cook with you or to enjoy a healthy new meal you have mastered. Avoid the fad or trend cookbooks in favor of cookbooks that stress the importance of fresh ingredients and only cook with healthy fats. Many healthy cookbooks will tell you the portion size and nutritional information of the suggested meal.

21. Teach a Child a New Sport

See the summer through the eyes of a young person. Make sure they have fun and ask them what are their favorite things about summer. Teach them a sport you played in your childhood or learn something new with them. Parents you are not off the hook. Even if you have the most athletic kids, try to find a new sport to enjoy together. You single guys and gals have no excuses either. If you don't have a niece or nephew, offer to baby-sit for a friend on a Saturday afternoon.

22. Host a Cookout and Replace Fatty Foods With Healthier Versions

You may be surprised by how tasty a turkey burger or even salmon burger can be. Increase the amount of lean protein in your diet without sacrificing the flavor or the social fun of a BBQ. Try grilling veggies and create a fruit salad for dessert. Invite your workout buddies to join in the fun. Healthy alternatives, such as salmon burgers can be found at grocery stores like Whole Foods or in the freezer section of your local market. These are just as tasty and offer a much healthier burger experience.

Think you will miss your burger? Consider this:

Burger	Calorie Count
Beef	511
Salmon	242
Turkey	150

Still think you'll miss that burger?

23. Map Out Three Different Walking or Jogging Paths

Find paths that all originate form your home. Make sure you can walk or jog for at least twenty minutes. The longer the course, the better. Find where they are, and plan to use all three this week.

The important thing is to get out in nature and enjoy it. If you are having a good time, you will workout longer and are more likely to do it. Start tracking your walks and jogs. See how far you can go and increase your pace and distance over time. You can try this one with your neighbor to increase your neighbor-to-neighbor bond.

24. Set a Weight-Loss Goal for Yourself Using Online Resources

Websites like www.AHA.org will help you determine your ideal weight and help plan how you can get there. Determine how many weeks it will take you to get to your ideal body weight losing two pounds a week. Do not start some scary fad diet or starve yourself. You are making lifelong changes. Losing two pounds a week is the healthy way to do it. We all know what happens when you set unrealistic goals or try to stick to diets that are too rigid and strict. Set-up a plan that you can stick to more easily. Have short-term and long-term goals that are appropriate.

Summer is a great time to lose weight because outdoor activities are popular and there are so many fresh fruit and vegetables available.

25. Do Not Check Your Email Before You Exercise

Don't miss workouts because you got caught up responding to email. You also don't want to be distracted during a workout by other things weighing on your mind. Read your emails when you have time to properly address them, not as you are running off to workout.

Protect your workout time. It is a commitment you have made to yourself. Treat your workout schedule like you would an important meeting.

26. Find a Committed Workout Partner

Working out can be more fun when you have a partner to keep you motivated. Post an ad on craigslist.org in your city or on a local community board. Ask around your office to see if a colleague will join you. Working out with a friend can help you de-stress and decrease your anxiety level, while at the same time motivate you to work out harder. A friend may also show you a few new exercises or give you a tip about proper form when lifting weights.

A workout partner is also someone who is depending on you to show up. If you have made plans to meet your workout partner, then you are committed and the chances that you will back out are much less.

Ideal Weight Tables For Men and Women

Ideal Weight For Women

Height in Shoes	Small Frame	Medium Frame	Large Frame
6'	138 to 151 lb	148 to 162 lb	158 to 179 lb
5'11"	135 to 148 lb	145 to 159 lb	155 to 176 lb
5'10"	132 to 145 lb	142 to 156 lb	152 to 173 lb
5'9"	129 to 142 lb	139 to 153 lb	149 to 170 lb
5'8"	126 to 139 lb	136 to 150 lb	146 to 167 lb
5'7"	123 to 136 lb	133 to 147 lb	143 to 163 lb
5'6"	120 to 133 lb	130 to 144 lb	140 to 159 lb
5'5"	117 to 130 lb	127 to 141 lb	137 to 155 lb
5'4"	114 to 127 lb	124 to 138 lb	134 to 151 lb
5'3"	111 to 124 lb	121 to 135 lb	131 to 147 lb
5'2"	108 to 121 lb	118 to 132 lb	128 to 143 lb
5'1"	106 to 118 lb	115 to 129 lb	125 to 140 lb
5'	104 to 115 lb	113 to 126 lb	122 to 137 lb
4'11"	103 to 113 lb	111 to 123 lb	120 to 134 lb
4'10"	102 to 111 lb	109 to 121 lb	118 to 131 lb

Ideal Weight For Men

Height in Shoes	Small Frame	Medium Frame	Large Frame
6'4"	162 to 176 lb	171 to 187 lb	181 to 207 lb
6'3"	158 to 172 lb	167 to 182 lb	176 to 202 lb
6'2"	155 to 168 lb	164 to 178 lb	172 to 197 lb
6'1"	152 to 164 lb	160 to 174 lb	168 to 192 lb
6'	149 to 160 lb	157 to 170 lb	164 to 188 lb
5'11"	146 to 157 lb	154 to 166 lb	161 to 184 lb
5'10"	144 to 154 lb	151 to 163 lb	158 to 180 lb
5'9"	142 to 151 lb	148 to 160 lb	155 to 176 lb
5'8"	140 to 148 lb	145 to 157 lb	152 to 172 lb
5'7"	138 to 145 lb	142 to 154 lb	149 to 168 lb
5'6"	136 to 142 lb	139 to 151 lb	146 to 164 lb
5'5"	134 to 140 lb	137 to 148 lb	144 to 160 lb
5'4"	132 to 138 lb	135 to 145 lb	142 to 156 lb
5'3"	130 to 136 lb	133 to 143 lb	140 to 153 lb
5'2"	128 to 134 lb	131 to 141 lb	138 to 150 lb

From height and weight tables of the Metropolitan Life Insurance Company, 1983. The ideal weights given in these tables are for ages 25 to 59. The weights assume you are wearing shoes with 1-inch heels and indoor clothing weighing 3 pounds.

HOW TO USE THE TIP PLANNERS

I have provided tips for each season. It is now your turn to incorporate these new healthy habits into your life. Begin keeping your records on the first day of the season. The first week of the season begins the Sunday following the first day of the season. I recommend filling in the dates of the weeks and then deciding on you vacation week first. This is your week break. You may decide to make this week coincide with an actual vacation, or perhaps it is the week you have out of town guest or perhaps it is just the week you want to be flexible.

Once you have set up your calendar, write down the corresponding number of the two tips you would like to do for that week. It is recommended to focus and commit to memory the tips you complete. Some seasons will have more body tips while some seasons will have more mind tips. Sprinkle in the fun tips to fill out all 13 weeks. Don't be afraid to double up on body tips on some weeks. The amount of each mind or body tip was determined by the desired focus for the particular season.

SUMMER TIPS PLANNER

Choose your two tips per week and place them under the heading, below called Tip #.

Put a line through each chosen tip after you have mastered it.

	Date	Tip #
Week 1	_____	_____
Week 2	_____	_____
Week 3	_____	_____
Week 4	_____	_____
Week 5	_____	_____
Week 6	_____	_____
Week 7	_____	_____
Week 8	_____	_____
Week 9	_____	_____
Week 10	_____	_____
Week 11	_____	_____
Week 12	_____	_____
Week 13	_____	_____

FEEL GOOD SUMMER TRACKER

Ideal Body Weight and Deviance +/- from the Ideal

Ideal Body Weight _____

June 21 _____
July weight *(within the 1st week)* _____
August weight *(within the 1st week)* _____
September weight *(within the 1st week)* _____

Total Calorie Intake Maintenance, Weight Loss, to Build Muscle
(your goals may change throughout the year, see www.feelgoodhealthnow.com)

Total Daily Calorie/Fat Gram/
    Protein Gram Intake for Maintenance _____
Total Daily Calorie/Fat Gram/
    Protein Gram Intake for Weight Loss _____
Total Daily Calorie/Fat Gram/
    Protein Intake to Build Muscle _____

Target Heart Rate for Aerobic Exercise
(see www.feelgoodhealthnow.com)

Moderate Intensity THR _____
High Intensity THR _____

FEEL GOOD SUMMER

Stressors: *(work, family, personal, financial or environmental)*
_____
_____
_____

Plan to cope with above stressors: _____
_____
_____
_____

Average Feel Good Score (1 to 10)
("1" is Completely Lousy and "10" is Blissful)

June 21	_____
July *(within the 1st week)* Date/Score	_____
August *(within the 1st week)* Date/Score	_____
September *(within the 1st week)* Date/Score	_____

Tips or life changes that increased your feel good score:
_____
_____
_____
_____
_____
_____
_____

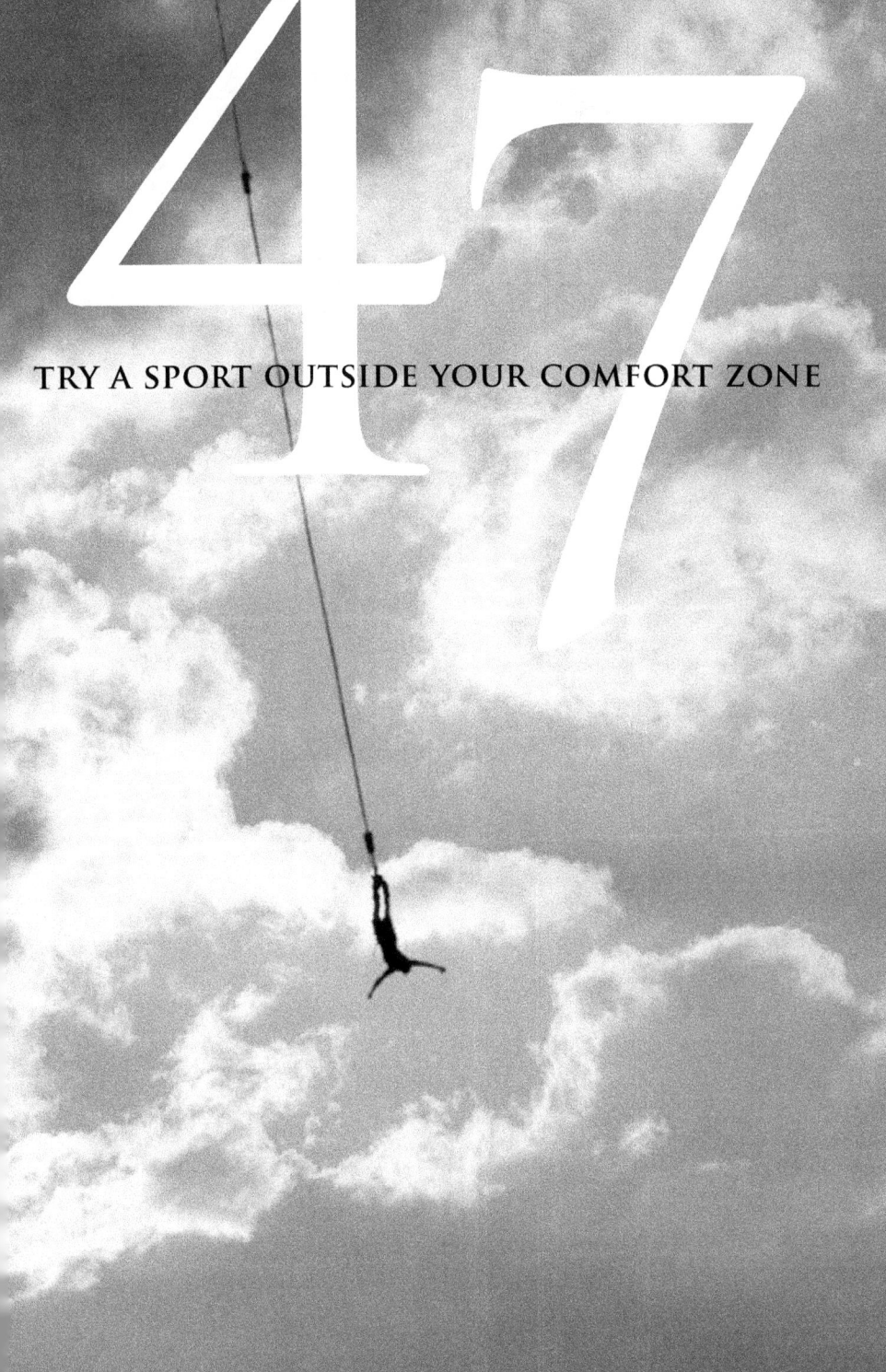

47

TRY A SPORT OUTSIDE YOUR COMFORT ZONE

FEEL GOOD FALL

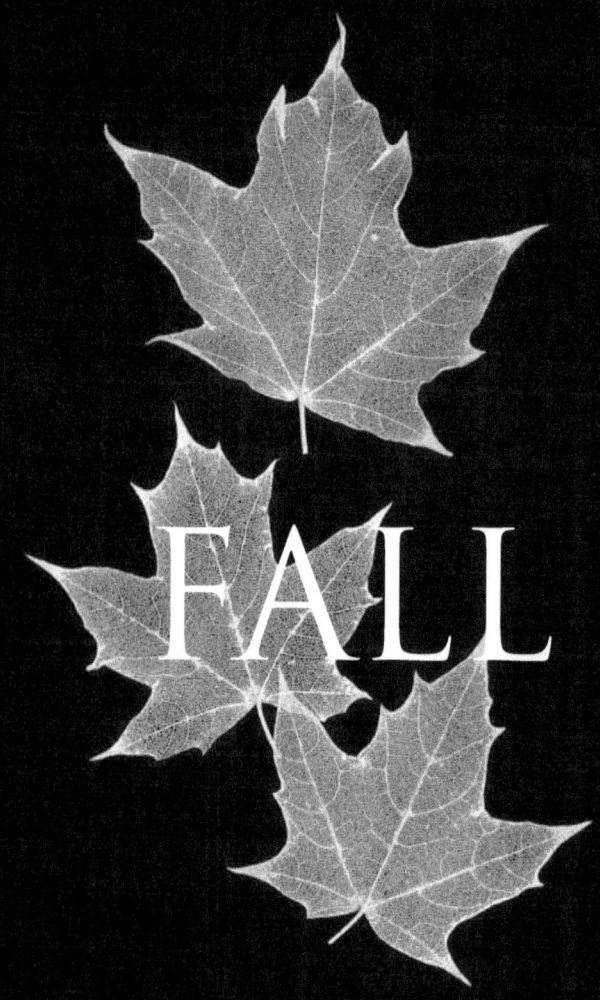

"The winds will blow their own freshness into you, and the storms their energy, while cares will drop off like autumn leaves."

– *John Muir*

GOALS FOR FALL

Stop Stress In Its Tracks:
Understand the genesis of stress and how to decrease your stressors at work and in your relationships. The tips this season will provide a guide to create happier interactions at work and at home.

Size Matters:
Learn and implement habits that will help you maintain a well-balanced and portioned diet. A good diet will give you more energy to make you feel and perform better.

You Must Diversify To Intensify:
Increase and diversify your aerobic and resistance training. This will prevent workout boredom and lead to the best side effect – a more fit and toned body. Along with that great body, it will energize your mind by "mixin it up" every once in awhile.

Doctor Shop Talk:
Learn how to talk to your doctor in order to get the most from your visits. It is important to you can relate your symptoms effectively and learn what screening tests (cholesterol levels, prostate and breast screenings) you should be getting.

FEEL GOOD FALL

The sweet summer wind has come and gone. Your summer fling has ended and now it's time to get serious. Well, maybe just more focused. There is no reason that the fun has to end. Autumn is a beautiful time of year and should be celebrated as much as summer was.

For me, fall has always been a time of excitement and apprehension. The end of summer means the start of a new academic year. When I was a kid, I could never sleep the night before the first day of a new school year. I was so excited to see friends that had left for the summer, but worried about new classes and new teachers.

Of all the seasonal changes, I found the change from summer to fall the most melancholy. I would always have this ache in my stomach that things were going to change. Moving from the security of a lazy summer to take on a greater academic challenge felt overwhelming. I experienced this stress starting in elementary school and then all throughout college and medical school.

However, I usually got tired of the lackadaisical summer attitude by mid-August and became anxious for the challenge of school. In fact, even though I was nervous, I welcomed the end of summer because I could only take so much of these do nothing summer days.

By the end of the summer, everyone seemed to have scattered out and were not a part of my life anymore. I was ready to see my friends again and have a structured and more stable life. Maybe you had enough of chumming around with your buddies and now it is time to get serious and start a meaningful relationship or put some more effort in your existing one.

Fall is a great time to get organized. While most of us are not going back to school this fall, we can still use fall as a time to re-evaluate the same things that students face. Are we dressed for success? Do we have all the tools we need to be successful in our lives this year? Are we ready to take on new challenges?

Just like going back to school, many things change for adults in the fall. Sometimes job changes occur, or we experience the anxiety of working more, or moving activities indoors as the weather grows colder.

We have to understand change and prepare for it, not just in a new job or academic situation, but in other life situations as well.

The people who handle stress the best are those who know it is coming and rehearse how to handle it so they can be mentally prepared. They can also be proactive about changing jobs, relationships or neighborhoods instead of reactive to such stresses. Do your best to avoid more than one of these major life changes at once, but stay prepared for the stress that these changes will present.

So what do you do when your job becomes increasingly stressful? One idea is to picture everyone at work that causes your stress in his or her underwear. Although admittedly there may be a co-worker you do not want to see in their underwear, and this might get complicated if you share this technique with co-workers. If the underwear trick does not work, I recommend a mental health day. Pick one day about every two weeks in which you get done with your major duties a few hours early. Either leave for a long lunch or take off a few hours early. I understand that many of us cannot leave work early. In that case, plan a decompress time at work. Offer to order in lunch for a few colleagues and take a break to enjoy each other's company, but don't talk about business.

Save a few vacation days and use one to try a new sport. Or take a vacation day to do something nice with your work support person or significant other. Americans do not always consider how much effort must be put into maintaining strong personal relationships.

Make sure that if you spend a lot of overtime at work one week, that the next week you shift the balance and make sure your significant other gets more attention. Occasionally, if we put as much time as we do in our 8 to 10 hour workdays for our significant other, friends, or family we would be awarded a substantial promotion of happiness.

Be flexible with your weekly schedule and make sure your personal relationships are getting the attention they deserve.

What Can You Do in the fall to Keep Active and Enrich the Lives of the People Around You?

What are the activities you did with your family and friends when you were young? Hiking through the forest? Taking a trip to a pumpkin patch to pick out a pumpkin and carve it for Halloween? Did you go out with your friends and family to trick or treat?

Halloween is always an exciting time for kids. Planning your costume, dressing up and what kid doesn't love all the free candy. I looked forward to it every fall when I was young. However, my father wanted to instill his hard work ethic in my four brothers and me. Before we could go trick-o-treating, we had to rake all of the leaves from our huge yard. I disliked, no I hated, raking leaves. My father was a taskmaster and had total disregard for what I thought were important child labor laws. We had to rake all the leaves into a massive pile and did I mention we had a really big yard? We did however, get to jump in them when we were done and I never missed a year of trick-o-treating. I know now that fall is a time to finish the hard chores so that we can all go out and play. Let Fall be a time of hard work and lots of fun.

A Few Suggestions For Fall Fun:

Try getting out on a bike tour. Find a country road or rural bike trail and go for a long bike ride with a friend or a group. If you are not a biker, then go for a long hike in the woods. Pack a lunch and make a day of it.

If you live near the coast, on either east or west coast, I recommend a scenic highway drive. Take mini trips to neighboring parks where they have social hiking groups that hunt for wild mushrooms, bird watch or geo-track.

Plan a trip to the wine country nearest you and take a walking or biking tour. If you have ever wanted to crush grapes between your feet, then fall is the best time to visit wine country. Wineries usually harvest in late September or early October. Fall is also apple-picking time. Visit an apple orchard where they feature a variety of apple trees. Do you know an orchard in Wisconsin has 120 different types of apples that you can sample? Some orchards have apple wine and fresh cider for tasting. Indulge, but not too much.

TIPS FROM THE M.D.

Health Benefits of Fiber

Fiber, fiber, fiber-everyone says eat more fiber and your mom said the same thing when she said, "Eat your vegetables." So, what is fiber? Fiber is a mostly indigestible substance found in the outer layers of plants. Fiber is a special type of carbohydrate that passes through the human digestive system virtually unchanged. You usually get the highest amount of fiber per serving when having the fruit or vegetable in its most natural form. For example, whole apples are a better source of fiber than applesauce and applesauce has more fiber than apple juice.

What foods are good sources of fiber? Whole grains, nuts, seeds, and legumes such as dried peas, beans, lentils, fruits and vegetables. Fiber is removed when foods are processed, so if you want to increase your fiber content, avoid processed foods.

If you do not think you are getting enough fiber, you can supplement it with a product like Metamucil, which when mixed with 8 ounces of water provides 4 to 6 grams of fiber.

Fiber absorbs increased water in the digestive tract, so stools are softer and easer to pass. A diet with adequate amounts of soluble fiber such as oats, rye barley, and beans helps to regulate cholesterol and decrease the risk of heart attack. Fiber in the diet helps to regulate blood sugar levels and can help in preventing the development of diabetes or may help control diabetes.

Fiber can also decrease the likelihood of developing diverticular disease, gallstones and kidney stones. Here is an added bonus, if fiber is taken at the right time and in sufficient quantities, fiber can slow the onset of hunger and help to control your weight.

Keep That Youthful Energy Through Fall:

Summer makes us all feel like little kids again. We play in the water, frolic in the park, and spend far too much time in the sun. How do we maintain the healthy youthful attitude into the fall? Let's first address your healthy, youthful image. Healthy is youthful. If you feel healthy, you feel youthful and vibrant.

Dress in clothes that make you feel comfortable and light. If you are to choose a jacket for autumn weather, choose one that is waterproof and lightweight. You should think about a windbreaker that has some warmth to it. Dress in clothes that make you feel young and vibrant. I am not suggesting that you pullout your old mini skirts, but dress in a flattering manner that makes you feel good. When you look good, you feel good. This positive attitude does wonders for your physical and mental health.

Now that you have the right attitude and clothes, let's work on your walk. Find ways to keep that spring in your step. It is said that you can tell a lot about a person by the way they walk. Do you have an efficient walk, a stern walk, or a youthful walk? What about how you sit or stand, and what about your posture? You can change these things.

No one taught us how to walk or sit, but maybe they should have. Just look at everyone's posture, really look around... terrible. Our posture has so much to do with how we feel and what aches and pains we experience. It also effects how others see us. In fact, many actors learn how to strut all over again using the Alexander technique. They learn how to walk in a more efficient, powerful and even youthful manner. There are many Alexander technique resources online and there are even teachers you can contact for advice. Now all you need to do is pick up a copy of Instyle Magazine, buy yourself a half-caf-non-fat-soy-latte and strut like the rest of Hollywood.

TIPS FROM THE M.D.

Dealing with Lower Back Pain

So you have not had the greatest posture for most of your life or you've had an accident or sports related injury and wound up with dreaded, lower back pain. Don't worry, you are not alone, four out of five adults experience low back pain at some point in their lives. There are several causes of low back pain; some of the more common causes include muscle strain, degenerative disc disease or lumbar herniated disc. The degree of pain in the lower back does not correlate with the cause of low back pain. You can have severe back pain with a muscle spasm and mild back pain with a significantly herniated disc. Your doctor will try to determine if you have weakness or numbness in your legs to determine if you have nerve compromise along with your back pain.

Treatment of low back pain depends on the cause. Muscle strains usually heal in a couple of days to several weeks. Exercise strengthens the core muscles that support the spine and can prevent the development of low back pain. The core muscles to strengthen include the back, abdominal and paraspinal or side muscles. Exercising these muscles will have the added benefit of improving your posture.

Low back pain that is worse in the morning and is associated with back stiffness is more characteristic of arthritis of the spine or osteoarthritis. Disc herniation is associated with pain or numbness that starts in the lower back and radiates down the leg. Low back pain associated with certain movements and positions is commonly caused by degenerative disc disease. Back exercises to strengthen the core muscles are beneficial for most types of back pain, but the cause of the back pain should be determined before any exercise or formal physical therapy begins.

Falls of the Past

Ah fall, a time of organization. Throughout recent and ancient history, fall is a time of harvest and regulation. To make sure we were all on time, at least on the same time, Greenwich established the universal time zones in the fall of 1884. These time zones were established on Midnight (GMT) October 13th to be exact. However, before we could worry about time we had to get everyone on the same date. Thus on October 4, 1582 the Gregorian calendar took effect. Once we had a reliable calendar we could set important dates, like Thanksgivings for example. Well, we would have to wait a few more centuries. The fall time festival was originally celebrated on December 4, 1619. It was not until Abraham Lincoln made it an official holiday, set on the last Thursday of November, that the country celebrated the day nationally. Franklin D. Roosevelt later moved the national day of over-eating to the fourth Thursday of the month.

Let's Talk Turkey

Turkey has many benefits and, in normal amount, is a great source of lean protein. Turkey also contains tryptophan, which in large quantities can put you to sleep faster than Uncle Pete's army stories. However, your post-meal sleepiness is more likely a result of massive overeating and not the tryptophan.

Do you know for a 2,000-calorie diet that we are only supposed to eat about 6 oz. of meat a day? Picture a standard deck of cards - this is about a 6 oz. portion. Seems small when you think of the average portion size we actually eat. You should also look at the other items on your plate. Just because you cut back on turkey doesn't mean that on Thanksgiving you should pile on more potatoes, stuffing, cranberry sauce, yams, and pumpkin pie.

Do you know the average size of the American plate in the year 1900 was about seven to nine inches in diameter? The current average is now eleven to twelve inches. That's only a couple of extra inches right? Wrong, eleven to twelve inches is only the diameter of the plate. Let's consider the area. Who remembers their geometry? The area of a 7-inch plate is 38.47 inches squared, and the 12-inch plate is 113.04 inches squared. That is nearly three times the area. Following that logic then we would be three times as fat, and sadly we are.

You do not have to fill every inch of your plate on Thanksgiving or at any meal. Just think about portion size when serving yourself. Sometimes it is difficult to know how big a portion is. Use standard objects to help remind your self. Your fist can be a great tool. Your fist represents one serving of salad, potatoes, and vegetables. Serving sizes of meats are generally a standard deck of cards. With foods such as oils, it is helpful to measure out how much you are using. Pretty soon you will get a feel for the look of a healthy portion of any item.

To make it easier here are some tricks. Find the salad plates in your set and use those as your dinner plate. Trick your eyes into thinking that you have a full plate. If you are more visual, mentally divide your plate into four sections. One section for protein, one for carbohydrates and the remaining two are for healthy fruits and vegetables.

TIPS FROM THE M.D.

Good and Bad Cholesterol

I am sure you have heard of good cholesterol and bad cholesterol by now. Often doctors will order a lipid panel to check your cholesterol levels. They are looking at four main lipids in your blood including triglycerides, and total cholesterol. Total cholesterol includes HDL (high-density lipoproteins, the good guys) and LDL (low-density lipoproteins, the bad guys).

If you have high total cholesterol or high levels of LDL, then you are at a greater risk for having heart attack and stroke. In general, if your cholesterol is over 200 or your LDL is greater than 100 you have risky cholesterol levels.

Why is one Cholesterol good and the other bad?
Cholesterol is not inherently bad; in fact it has important functions in the body. Cholesterol is responsible for making and maintaining cell membranes, making sex hormones, producing vitamin D and it also aides digestion by making bile salts.

Unfortunately, high levels cholesterol will speed up the process know as atherosclerosis. This is the process of putting lipid layers on the inside of the blood vessel, which can lead to the clotting of a vessel. If the blocked vessel leads to the heart it can cause a heart attack. If the blocked vessel leads to the brain it can cause stroke.

LDL (the bad stuff) is responsible for lining blood vessels and causing atherosclerosis. Many factors within our control will lead to higher LDL cholesterol levels. These factors include a diet high in fat, smoking, diabetes, and high blood pressure.

The HDL (the good stuff) circulates around the blood vessels and extracts floating (bad) cholesterol before it can be deposited on the blood vessel. Exercise can increase your HDL level.

Nutrition Facts

I strongly recommend mypyramid.gov for learning about your personal nutritional needs. This site breaks down your diet and provides recommendations for how much of each food group you should be eating.

For example, for a 30-year-old woman, 5 ft. 5 in., who is physically active less than 30 minutes a day, the recommended amounts of each category are:

Vegetables	2.5 cups
Fruits	2 cups
Grains *(half should be whole grains)*	6 ounces
Milk	3 cups
Meat and Beans	5.5 ounces
Oils	6 teaspoons
Total Calories	2,000
Discretionary Calories	265

For a 30 year old man, 5 ft. 9 in. tall, and is physically active less than 30 minutes a day, the recommended amounts of each category are:

Vegetables	3 cups
Fruits	2 cups
Milk	3 cups
Meat and Beans	6.5 ounces
Oils	7 teaspoons
Total Calories	2,400
Discretionary Calories	360

Discretionary calories are extra fats and sugars.

The vegetables should be varied from dark green, *(spinach and other leafy greens)*, to orange *(carrots, sweet potatoes, and pumpkin)*, and include dry beans, peas and starches such as corn, potatoes, green beans.

Autumn Cocktail:

   4 part Good Nutrition
   1 part Hard Work
   3 parts Preparation and Organization
   2 parts Family and Friend Time

Muddle ingredients together until hard work and fun are infused. Sip slowly. Best enjoyed while carving pumpkins or picking apples.

The Dreaded Yearly Physical

Okay, so you overdid it on Thanksgiving because it was just so good and you did not want to insult your Aunt Jenny when she insisted you have a third piece of sweet potato pie. Now you need to check out the damage. It is a perfect time to visit your doctor for your yearly physical.

I know going to the doctor can be down right scary, but taking the time to assess what's going on now can prevent underlying issues from festering into something serious.

Let me take some of the mystery out of the doctor's office and give you some tips on making your visit less painful and more productive. First of all, bring all your medicine bottles with you when you visit the doctor. Don't try to remember the names, most of them sound a like and your doctor can learn a lot by knowing what dosage you are on. Also make sure you bring any discharge forms the hospital or clinic and any lab or X-ray reports. Doctors love this stuff and the more the better. Expect the doctor to ask a lot of questions.

When doctors do a physical, they are always very interested in your vital signs, pulse, blood pressure, respirations and temperature.

You should ask your doctor what screening test you need. Your doctor can discuss with you, based on your test results, how frequently you should have a blood profile and other screening tests. Screening for breast, prostate, colon and other types of cancers are important for early detection. Your doctor will advise you, based on your condition, how frequently you should be checked.

Conditions such as diabetes, high blood pressure and heart disease will merit more frequent visits. Be sure to discuss with your doctor how often you need to make appointments.

TIPS FROM THE M.D.

The Flu Shot

Should I get the flu shot? Yes.
 There are millions of strains of viruses in existence, but only a few grow strong enough each year to wreak havoc on your body. Every year, the Center for Disease Control (CDC) puts together the flu shot to protect us from the viral strains they think will be the major players in the upcoming year. The side effects include the possibility of a low-grade fever, lasting twenty-four to forty-eight hours, and general malaise. Just think about it - if it were not safe, then why is it given out at schools.

 The flu shot is very beneficial for the elderly. Thousands of elderly die each year of the flu or flu related complications. Many elderly get pneumonia, an infection in the lungs that can lead to death. A small shot seems worth avoiding nasty infections, days cooped up in bed, and possible death.

 In addition to warding off the flu, fall brings up other issues. After a summer of hanging out in the sun, you wake up one morning to find that there are new wrinkles on your face. Do you immediately run to the phone and call your local plastic surgeon or dermatologist? Stop, there is no reason to call in the big guns. Remember that your primary care doctor can make you look and feel good inside and out, so don't forget about us. If you absolutely must call the plastic surgeon make sure you choose a surgeon who has a lot of experience with the procedure. Be sure to check their credentials. Ask them to explain the risks and the recovery in detail. You might want to talk to some of their previous patients.

FALL INTO HEALTH TIPS

27. Buy a New CD or Download Music That Provides a Calming Effect

Let's face it, once fall turns cold we will be spending more time indoors or in our cars. Make this transition more peaceful by learning to relax. Soothing music can help you take the stress out of an unpleasant situation. Learn to sit still and enjoy the calming effect of your new music.

28. Go For a Fall Bike Ride

Fall is a beautiful time of year because the bitter cold of winter has not set in and the harsh heat of summer is a thing of the past. Use this time of year to get outside as much as possible. Take a bike ride through a neighborhood where you can enjoy the fall foliage. Keep your eye on the road, but don't forget to experience all the wonderful colors of fall. Get a few friends together or take your family out for a bike ride one afternoon. If it is getting cold, pack some hot apple cider or hot chocolate and enjoy the fall scenery.

29. Focus On Time Management and Take Note of All the Redundant and Unnecessary Things You Do In a Day

The days are getting shorter and the kids are going back to school. Even if you don't have kids, everyone notices a return to more normal routines in the fall. The lazy days of summer are over and time is of the essence. This is a great season to work on your time management skills. Spend a few moments with your day planner each morning to review what tasks and events you have for the day. Plan times when you can rest and when you need to be particularly active. A few minutes in the morning will help you organize your whole day and prevent you from missing deadlines or forgetting important events. At the end of the day, reflect back on your busy day. Was there a period when you wasted a lot of time? Are you constantly late because your morning television show slows you down? Does checking your email every fifteen minutes distract you from important work projects? Find ways to get back your time. Taking small steps to improve the efficacy of your work will give you extra time to workout or spend quality time with your friends and family.

30. Replace Your Coffee Break With a 15-Minute Walk To Get Out of the Office

Yes, the lunch hour has gotten shorter and breaks are harder to come by, but even short breaks will do you a world of good. Find ways to get out of the office, even if you just walk down to the lobby. Getting out and walking is great for your body, especially if you sit at a desk all day. Walk over to a co-worker to plan a meeting instead of sending an email. Taking a few minutes to walk around will also help you focus better. You will be surprised how refreshed you feel after stepping away from the computer screen even for a moment. If you need coffee on your coffee break, don't walk to the closest Starbucks, walk to the one a few blocks further away.

31. Try To Identify With One Past Emotional Trauma To Start the Process of Coming To Terms With It

We have heard of the terms battle fatigue, shell shock, or Post Traumatic Stress Disorder (PTSD). All of these terms relate to past events, the first two more relate to past military experiences and the emotional aftermath. Subconsciously, we may all have a number of past events and are still experiencing lingering effects of the trauma now. We may have had a bad experience at the dentist and now get anxious every time we go, hence instead of going to the dentist every 6 months, it has been 2 years.

We may have many of these past traumas that linger. Take a moment to reflect on your stresses on your mind. Is it something that happened recently or is something that happened in the past and is still lingering. Becoming fully aware of these stresses is the first step in dealing with them and becoming more at peace.

32. Adopt the TRAF (Trash, Refer, Act, and File) System To File Any Papers That Come Across Your Desk or Your Email Inbox

Think about your desk, at home or at your office. What condition is it in? Most of us have trouble keeping up with all the paperwork and emails that we receive each day. Things are lost or forgotten and the "to do" stack keeps growing. These little things add up to a whole lot of stress. They weigh on your mind at inopportune times- like when you are trying to sleep. When you receive paperwork or read a new email, decide if you need to trash it, refer or forward the information, act on it, or file it for review later. This simple organizational system will help you keep on top of things at work and at home. It might even help you sleep better at night.

33. Do Something For Yourself To Improve Your Self-Esteem

All too often we reward ourselves with food, a nice dinner, a good bottle of wine, or a giant candy bar. However, these things don't last and neither does the good feeling they temporarily provide. Instead of eating, try buying a nice pair of shoes or paying a little extra for a special style and haircut. A nice dinner can cost the same as a day at the spa. If your budget is a little tight, try getting a massage at a training school or give yourself a facial at home. Find ways to pamper yourself and feel good.

34. Take a Mental Health Day Off Work and Spend Time With the People In Your Support Network

Many offices are now realizing that their employees need mental health time off. If you have been stressed out or if your home life is feeling overwhelming, take a day off to catch-up. Run all your errands early so that you have time to meet with friends for lunch or surprise your child at school. You can use this day to try a new sport with your friends or practice a new skill together. Make sure to spend time with your family or invite your friends over for a small get together. Use this time off to show your support network that you appreciate them and support them.

35. Identify Your Financial Stresses and Develop a Long-Term Plan to Deal With Them

When I talk with my patients, we identify different categories of stress: situational, work related, family and parenting and financial. All of these stresses can affect us and bring us down but it seems like financial stress is a category unto itself that needs to be dealt with differently. Financial stresses affect our health in different ways. We worry about finances and our body experiences all the affects of stress.

Financial stress can cause worsening interpersonal problems. Financial concerns are the number two reason people break up. Communication is the number one reason people split. Do not feel isolated; talk to friends and family who are better with financial information to get you back on your feet.

36. Try These Meditation Websites and Put Your Own Music To the Meditation

Meditation does not have to be hard. You don't even need to go to some center and sit on brightly colored mats to meditate. There are several resources you can use from home. Find a guided meditation CD or podcast and try the meditation regimen at home or work. There are also websites that give visual images to view while meditating. Try this one on for size: http://www.myss.com/vismed.asp# There are several more available on the Internet. Find one that works best for you.

37. Learn the Proper Portions for Fruits and Vegetables

Most of us have heard that we need five serving of fruits and vegetables each day. Some sources even recommend five to nine servings a day. However, most of us do not get nearly the right amount. Work on increasing the amount of dark green and orange vegetables or fruits in your diet. Have a small salad before dinner so that you fill up on good for you veggies before you think about going for seconds on less healthy options. Crave sweets after a savory meal? Cut up some fruits or serve berries for dessert. You may find that they do the trick and you really don't need that bowl of ice cream. How much is a portion? On average a piece of fruit is a serving. Think about an average sized apple. For veggies it is about a fist size. Over the course of a whole day I'm sure you can eat five fist sizes of fruits and vegetables.

38. On Your Next Visit To Your Doctor, Ask Them About Prevention Medicine For Your Age Group

Become aware of the normal screening procedures. Screening procedures are tests designed to pick up disease in the population and are based on probabilities of getting a certain medical condition for your age and sex. Many do not want to visit the doctor because they are afraid that they may be told some bad health news or the doctor is going to get on you for having bad habits, such as smoking. I tell my patients I am here to support you, not nag you, but I am going to remind you every time about your weight. Blood pressure should be checked annually. In general, after age 20 a cholesterol panel should be checked every 5 years or every 2 years if you have heart or stroke risk factors.

To detect colon cancer, all adults should have a colonoscopy, where there look "up" your colon, at age 50 and then at least every 10 years. Women should in general have a PAP smear yearly to detect cervical cancer and a mammogram every 1 to 2 years starting at age 50, earlier if there are symptoms or if they have a relative that has been diagnosed with breast cancer. Men over 50 should get a PSA, a blood test, to detect prostate cancer.

39. Drink Plenty of Water

About 70% of the earth is covered with water. We are made up of about the same amount of water. There must be something to this water thing. Well there is. You can go several days without food and still recover, but just a few days without water and we are talking about organ failure and total body shut down.

Yes, you really do need eight, 8 oz. glasses of water a day. The body needs water to function properly and if you are trying to lose weight, good luck doing it without the proper hydration. The body looses water all day long from more than just sweating and urination. Did you know the lungs expel between two and four cups of water a day?

Measure how much water you need and make sure you are drinking that each day. Eight, 8 oz. glasses is 1.9 liters. That is about the size of a two-liter Coke bottle.

You need to drink even more water if you are in hot weather, sick, or breastfeeding.

40. Identify the Communication Blocks and Questions For Your Doctor

I know doctors can be intimidating. They use big words, order weird tests, and sometimes forget what language the rest of us speak. Trust me, your doctor wants only the best for you, but sometimes communication can be frustrating. Before you go to the doctor review your medical history and make sure you take your prescription and over the counter medications with you. Write down your questions and take a pad of paper and a pen with you. Make sure you get all your questions answered and write down information you don't want to forget.

If you don't understand something or if your doctor is using a term you are not familiar with, stop them and ask. Doctors spend most of their undergraduate years studying science and then spend four years in medical school learning about your medical issue.

My point is that they have at least eight years of knowledge on you, but do not feel stupid or silly if you have a lot of questions. Doctors can be notoriously difficult to get a hold off, so make sure your questions are answered while you are in the appointment room.

Often people will look up their symptoms online before coming in or check out their condition in a chat room. I always recommend that my patients educate themselves. What doctor doesn't love an educated patient? However, don't get tunnel vision. Don't think that the Internet has provided you with the end-all-be-all diagnosis and treatment for what ails you. Keep an open mind and collaborate with your doctor.

41. Check Your Posture Out and Here Are Some Exercises to Improve Your Posture

Sit up straight! We have all heard this at some point in our lives. However, there is a lot more to proper posture than just sitting correctly. Posture has to do with how we sit, stand, walk, and lay down. When we stand or walk with proper posture, the least amount of strain is placed on the supporting muscles and ligaments. Proper posture leads to the following: bones and joints that are in proper alignment, decreased wearing of joint surfaces, and decreased stress on ligaments. Good posture will also prevent abnormal spine positioning, fatigue, backache, and muscle pain. Best of all, if you walk with good posture you will have an over all good appearance.

It is hard to judge our own posture, but check out resources about posture and ask a friend to watch you walk. You can also get a posture or walking coach. Your walk says a lot about you and effects how you feel. It's worth spending some time evaluating your posture.

42. Buy Fresh, Dried, Frozen and Canned Fruits (In Water or Juice) So They Are Always Available

Think fresh fruits are healthier than frozen bagged goods? Well, not always. If you could pick the fruits fresh from your back yard or even buy them from the farmer's market then, absolutely, fresh is best. However, when you factor in travel time, shelf time at the grocery store, and the time the fruits sit in your refrigerator, then hands down frozen wins every time. While fresh fruits are loosing their nutrients, frozen fruits are frozen as soon as they are picked. This preserves the nutrients, and no, freezing does not destroy cell walls. Ranked in the order of most healthy: Frozen is best when fruit has to travel far, fresh is better if you are picking the fruit yourself. Canned fruits fall slightly behind and are definitely last if the fruit is drenched in high fructose corn syrup. Dried fruits are great too, if they are eaten in moderation. Beware of portion distortion. With all the water removed, dried fruit has the same amount of calories for much smaller portions. In whatever form, make sure you are enjoying your fruits.

43. Learn the Differences Between Overweight and Obese and Find Out Where You Stand

To define both we must first learn about Body Mass Index (BMI). BMI is a measure of body fat based on your height and weight. It is the same for men and women. Your BMI score will place you in one of four categories:

Underweight =	<18.5
Normal Weight =	18.5 – 24.9
Overweight =	25 – 29.9
Obesity =	BMI of 30 or greater

Overweight refers to an increase in body weight in relation to your height when compared to the desired weight for a person of equal height. Obesity is defined as an excessively high amount of body fat in relation to lean body mass. Many health risks are associated with obesity, including "http://en.wikipedia.org/wiki/Cardiovascular_diseases"cardiovascular diseases, diabetes, "http://en.wikipedia.org/wiki/Sleep_apnea"sleep apnea, and "http://en.wikipedia.org/wiki/Osteoarthritis"osteoarthritis.

According to clinical studies, if you have a BMI of over 25, then you are putting your health at risk. Don't let these numbers discourage or depress you, instead use this as a motivation to get out there and get active, eat better, and stay on top of your tips each season.

44. Have At Least 5 Servings of Fruits and Vegetables a Day

This is a hard one for most Americans, but it is so good for you and truly one of the best ways to maintain a healthy diet. First, fruits and vegetables are usually fat-free, low-cal and packed with essential vitamins, nutrients, and the all-important fiber. Vegetables will leave you feeling full longer and fruits can curb a post-meal sweet tooth. Find fun ways to include fruits and veggies into each meal. Use difference spices or incorporate vegetables into your favorite pasta dishes. Make sure you have a small salad with dinner or make a hearty salad your dinner. Take fruits to work as an afternoon pick-me-up or make a fruit salad for dessert. Drink fruit or vegetable juices but watch your portion sizes. Juices can be a great way to get your five on the run, but juices can have more calories without the fiber of the actual fruit or vegetable.

45. Be a Guest at Your Friend's Health Club or Try a Free Lesson at the Local Health Club

Many health clubs will let you test-out their facilities for a couple of days, or even a week if you show interest. Gyms are always giving their members free passes. Check with one of your gym-rat friends, chances are they have extra guest passes lying around. Scope out a few gyms and find one that makes your feel comfortable and motivates you to workout. There are gyms for men, women, families and various sports all over. If you are going to workout three to five times a week, make sure your gym is a place you want to be. If the annual cost of membership is a little daunting, check with your local YMCA. They often have low cost membership for gym use, classes, and athletic teams.

46. Do a Friend-Building Activity with Your Support Friend

Leaving the very social season of summer behind, fall is a great time to start establishing a stronger support network. Plan one-on-one times with your friends. Instead of getting dinner, or grabbing drinks, try a different bonding experience. Do an act of charity or spend an afternoon working with underprivileged kids. Prepare a healthy meal together or offer to help a friend with a project that is hanging over their head. You will need their support in the future so make sure that you are there for your support network when they need you.

47. Try a Sport Outside Your Comfort Zone

Time to get brave and step outside your safety zone. Go bouldering, rock climbing, skydiving, or swing on a trapeze. Maybe you haven't ridden a bike in years and that sounds risky to you. Just get out there and do something new. Why test your comfort zone? Well, because it is important to test yourself. Don't get stuck in a routine and forget to be adventurous. The adrenaline rush alone is energizing and makes you feel more alive. Even better is the confidence that comes when you step out of your comfort zone and accomplish what you set out to do.

48. Take a Weekend Get Away and Lie in the Grass and Look Up at the Stars and the Moon

Life is hectic. Regardless of where you live, there are modern-day stressors and stress triggers all around you. Plan a weekend get away where you leave your troubles behind. You don't have to go far or pick the most exciting destination. Just get away and relax. Of course, take your cell phone in case of emergencies but don't check your email. Stay at a bed and breakfast. They are cozy, relaxing and usually less expensive than a traditional hotel.

49. Use Protein Bars, Shakes, and Smoothies as Food to Increase Your Alertness and Focus

Everyone is on the run these days. When are we supposed to find the time to prepare three healthy, protein-packed meals each day? Protein is so important for concentration and energy. If you don't have time to prepare a healthy lunch or if you get stuck eating lunch in the office each day, then try a protein bar or shake. They are a quick and easy way to get the nutrients your body needs. Just watch your calories. Most of these bars and shakes are meal replacement size and should not be eaten as snacks.

50. Next Time You Order Pizza, Order a Healthy Pizza

There will always be days when you feel like you have been run over by a truck and ordering a pizza feels like the only sane option. Eating pizza every once and a while is fine, but make the pizza as healthy as possible. If you are a double cheese meat lover's fanatic, try to scale it back a bit. Pizza meats are high in saturated fats and are loaded with salt. Ask your pizzeria if they offer chicken, shrimp or another healthy alternative. Find vegetables you enjoy and ask for light cheese. Trust me, you will feel better and will be more mentally equip to handle the stress of your day if you eat a healthier pizza.

51. Try Power or Speed Walking

Summer is for casual strolls, but now it is getting cold outside and it is time to pick up the pace. Walking has great health benefits and best of all it is free. The average person walks about 3 miles per hour. This is just slightly faster than a stroll. To speed walk you have to get those feet moving and your heart beating faster. Power walking is when you walk a twelve-minute mile or up to five miles an hour. Speed walking is walking at a pace over five miles per hour. No matter what your current athletic condition, you can walk. The more you do it, the faster you will be able to go.

52. Take Ten-Minute Turns Actively Listening to Your Significant Other Every Day

Many couples say one of the most important reasons that they stay together so long is that they continue to really talk to each other. Poor communication is the number one reason people divorce. In my medical practice, I see the myriad of mental and physical problems that develop from people who are isolated and alone. Get connected, really connected. People are both going to grow individually, but as long as individuals share some of their growth they have better chance of making it. The good news is that if you are both good listeners, you can take the relationship to new levels of trust and greater heights of intimacy. Quite frankly, everyone likes to be heard. Positive attention makes us feel good.

FALL TIPS PLANNER

Choose your two tips per week and place them under the heading, below called Tip #.

Put a line through each chosen tip after you have mastered it.

	Date	Tip #
Week 1		
Week 2		
Week 3		
Week 4		
Week 5		
Week 6		
Week 7		
Week 8		
Week 9		
Week 10		
Week 11		
Week 12		
Week 13		

FEEL GOOD FALL TRACKER

Ideal Body Weight and Deviance +/- from the Ideal

Ideal Body Weight _____

September 23 _____
October weight *(within the 1st week)* _____
November weight *(within the 1st week)* _____
December weight *(within the 1st week)* _____

Total Calorie Intake Maintenance, Weight Loss, to Build Muscle
(your goals may change throughout the year, see www.feelgoodhealthnow.com)

Total Daily Calorie/Fat Gram/
    Protein Gram Intake for Maintenance _____
Total Daily Calorie/Fat Gram/
    Protein Gram Intake for Weight Loss _____
Total Daily Calorie/Fat Gram/
    Protein Intake to Build Muscle _____

Target Heart Rate for Aerobic Exercise
(see www.feelgoodhealthnow.com)

Moderate Intensity THR _____
High Intensity THR _____

FEEL GOOD FALL

Stressors: *(work, family, personal, financial or environmental)*
_____
_____
_____

Plan to cope with above stressors: _____
_____
_____
_____

Average Feel Good Score (1 to 10)
("1" is Completely Lousy and "10" is Blissful)

September 23	_____
October *(within the 1st week)* Date/Score	_____
November *(within the 1st week)* Date/Score	_____
December *(within the 1st week)* Date/Score	_____

Tips or life changes that increased your feel good score:
_____
_____
_____
_____
_____
_____
_____

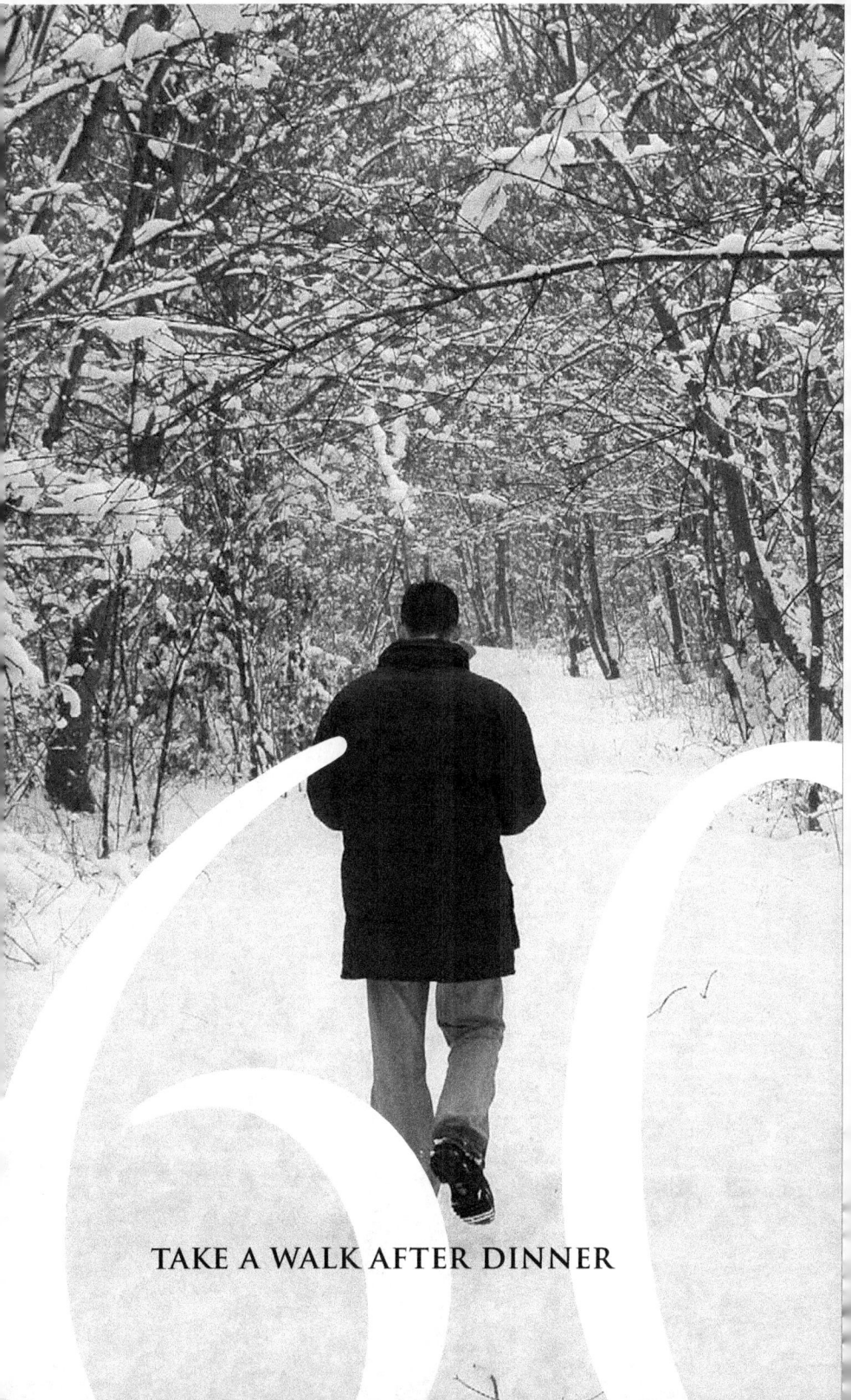

FEEL GOOD WINTER

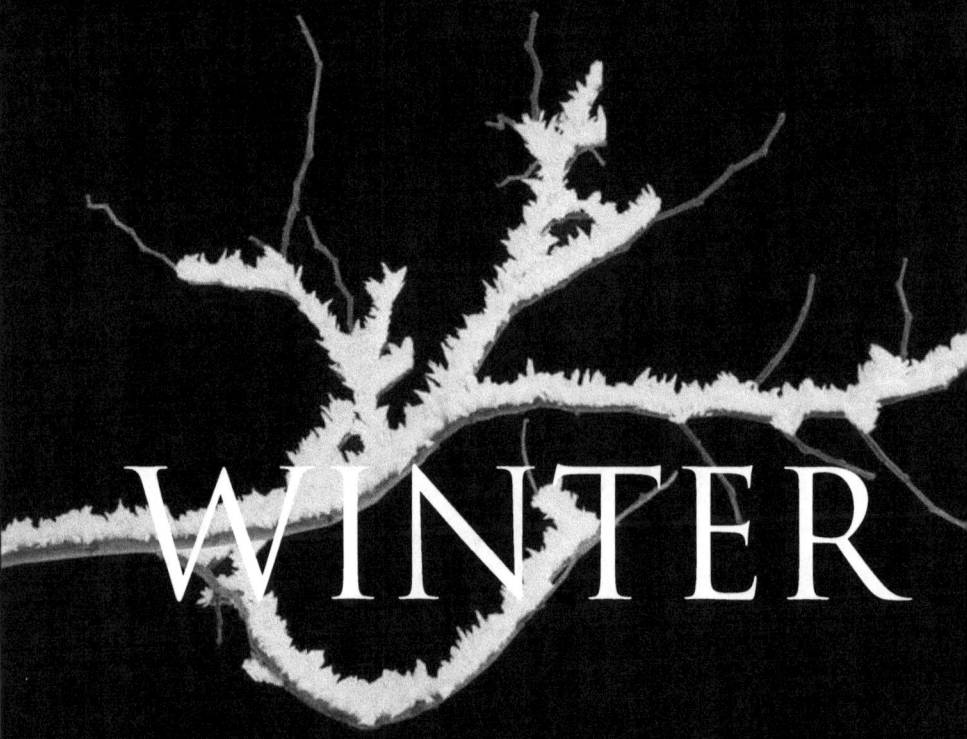

WINTER

"Laughter is the sun that drives winter from the human face."

– *Victor Hugo*

GOALS FOR WINTER

Snowed In Games:
To cope with the stresses of winter, including the decreasing light in the day, isolation and hibernation, develop a hardy attitude to prevent cabin fever, anxiety and depression.

Put a Cap in Your Sweet Tooth:
Become aware of the type and amount of fats and sweets that you consume in a day and the fat and sweet substitutes. I will show you how to lower your bad cholesterol and raise your good cholesterol.

No Membership Required:
Learn how to set-up your home gym in the bedroom or the TV room to help with your flexibility, resistance (weight training) and aerobic goals at home. You can pace yourself at home and the health club so your New Year's resolution does not become your New Year's embarrassment.

Gazuntight:
Be able to recognize the symptoms and signs of a cold, the flu, bronchitis and pharyngitis. Learn ways to strengthen your immune system and decrease the occurrence of these pesky maladies.

FEEL GOOD WINTER

Popcorn Tins, Candy Dishes and Cookies Everywhere! They come earlier and earlier every year. Holiday tins of cookies, candies and cakes. They just keep coming. They are everywhere around the office and they're in your dining and living room. Become aware of these tempters. The classic tin of popcorn contains the triple threat: butter, cheese and caramel. The caramel corn has the higher fat and calories so go easy on these carmal delites. For this six to eight week holiday period, you need to be extra conscientious and have a fat and sweet allowance.

Visit mypyramid.gov to find out what your daily cheat allowance would be. If you are going for the snacks, focus on smaller portions and the nuts. Actually the popcorn is a good source of fiber, so have a few more of the lightly buttered or cheese stuff and less of the caramel corn. Nuts or seeds are healthy for you as well. However, I am sure you have heard, avoid the bad trans fats and eat more of the good polyunsaturated and monounsaturated fats. During the holidays, there is plenty of bad trans fat guys around. You need to just get in the habit of thinking about everything you put in your mouth during this snacks-abound season.

Daily Sweet Allowance

While it is nearly impossible to completely avoid sweets and some junk food during the holidays, it is important to know how much you can indulge.

On a daily basis, your total snack allowance should be about 200 to 300 calories, 70 calories from fat (check-varies for each individual). Below is a list of the foods with the number of calories per snack. If you do indulge beyond that, take the snack trays away the next day. If it gets out of control, take an alternate route around the snack sites in the office and only have the snack trays out at home when company comes.

Cookies:	260 calories -	11 fat grams
Carmel corn:	141 calories -	10 fat grams
Cheese popcorn:	58 calories -	3.7 fat grams
Buttered popcorn:	97 calories -	7.8 fat grams *(not movie theater)*
Peanuts:	166 calories -	14.1 fat grams
Peppermints:	59 calories -	0 fat grams

Stick to your sweet and fat allowance because it all adds up through the course of the winter.

TIPS FROM THE M.D.

Just What Actually Happens When You Eat That Chocolate Caramel Vs. Some Toasted Almonds?

Chocolate and caramel are comprised of simple sugars and are metabolized in about an hour, whereas nuts contain good fats that are broken down and in our blood stream in about 3 to 4 hours in a more sustained way. Basically, the nuts will keep you full longer and will provide more energy. The chocolate and caramel are quickly broken down and more readily stored as fat.

Home Gyms Vs. Health Clubs

I recommend a gym membership at a health club. It is a great place to work out, be social, and get advice.

How do you get the most out of your health club?
First, get a good tour. Learn how to use every machine by asking a trainer or a fellow workout partner; they might teach you a new trick or two to keep you from getting bored.

If you have the space, you can set up a weight or cardio station at home. The best place to host a weight set and cardio room in your home is in the ground level or basement. The room should be about 12ft by 10ft. You need a bench (cost aprox. $120) and a basic 110lb. to 300lb. weight set ($150 to $200) and a mat you can do stretching or yoga on.

If you have the resources, have a certified personal trainer come to your house to be involved in the set up and at least the first few sessions. Some people have personal trainers come to their homes

2 to 3 times a week. A personal trainer with good nutrition knowledge can be very helpful at your home because they can take a look in your frig and recommend some wellness food options.

Don' worry if you can't convert an entire room into your personal gym, there are plenty of other options. If you spend a lot of time in front of the TV, try to set up a resistance training and flexibility area. Ideally, you should have a gym plan and a home plan. It is harder to get out in the winter, but if you are set up at home with the right technique or dumbbells your can get in a good workout during a show.

We need to pace ourselves for a potentially long winter. Activities outside the home should not stop. I will help you with some strategies to remain active mentally and physically.

Winter Sports - Both Outdoor and Indoor

So winter is here, but the sports don't have to stop. There are indoor golf driving ranges, tennis courts, racquetball, and indoor climbing and boldering walls for the more adventurous. When I was young, after a heavy snowfall, my four brothers and I would build a bobsled track, complete with banked curves. Go out of your comfort zone and learn how to ski or snowboard, if you have not already mastered both. You will be surprised at your proficiency down the bunny slopes or maybe the intermediate slopes by the end of the day.

TIPS FROM THE M.D.

'Tis the Season for Cold and Flu's

How Can You Tell These Two Apart and What To Do When You Get These

So just what is the difference between a cold and the flu? Well, a virus causes both colds and the flu. A low-grade fever and muscle and joint aches usually accompany both as well. A specific virus called Influenza causes the flu. The course for the flu is usually longer and can lead to more severe dehydration.

So why do we get more colds in the winter? It is actually because we are indoors more and thus exposed to others somewhat more. With a strong immune system, it is much harder to catch a cold. Do things that strengthen and improve your immune system, like getting enough sleep.

A virus called rhinovirus causes the common cold. There are about 200 types of rhinoviruses, all of which are very diverse. Since they are so diverse, a vaccine is not possible.

How do doctors determine if you have a cold (caused by a virus) or a bacterial infection (bronchitis, sinusitis)? Usually a cold causes a low-grade fever temperature between about 99F and 100.5F and a bacterial infection has a fever between 100.5F and above.

What Do You Do If You Have a Cold?

Do you starve a cold and feed a fever? No, and I'm not even sure where that logic came from. If you do get a cold there are substances that help our immune system. Medical research in the last few decades shows some benefit of zinc lozenges to reduce the duration and severity of the common cold symptoms. Just about every culture around the world embraces the concept that chicken soup helps soothe the cold. Yes, I definitely think there is something soothing about chicken soup, especially mom's homemade recipe.

You Tried Every Way To Avoid It But You Got the Flu

First of all just, what is the flu and how is it different from a cold. The Influenza virus can be treated by antiviral medications, unlike the common cold. Typically in a doctor's office, there is a nasal swab to detect the different strains of Influenza A, B or C.

You need to take the antiviral medication within 2 days of being sick. Depending on the type of Influenza virus that you contract, the antiviral medication may be more or less effective. The antiviral medications reduce the symptoms and may shorten the time you are sick by one to two days.

Symptoms of the flu include fever (usually high), headache, tiredness, a sore throat and a dry cough, body and or joint aches and nasal congestion. The Influenza virus is spread from person to person, primarily through droplet transmission (e.g. when an infected person coughs or sneezes in a close proximity to an uninfected person).

How long are you infectious to others? You can be infectious the day before symptoms arise and 5 days after the onset of the illness.

The people who are at high risk for the flu are people 65 years or older, people with chronic heart and lung conditions, pregnant women, and young children.

Here are a few strategies for preventing the flu that the Center for Disease Control (CDC) recommends. First, avoid close contact with people who are sick and stay at home if you are sick. Cover your mouth and nose when you cough or sneeze and yes, wash your hands for about 15 to 20 seconds, the time it takes you to sing the ABC song. Avoid touching your eyes, nose and mouth. Practice lifestyle tips to keep your immune system at its peak-get enough sleep, limit stress, and drink plenty of fluids

Winter Depth

Winter can be a tough time if you live in less temperate climates. We tend to read more, watch more television, and spend less time out with friends. There is less outside interaction and more time for deep reflection. Reflection is a good thing, but too much reflection can lead to cabin fever. Depression or dysthymia, a milder chronic form of depression, can set in when obsessions continue to fester and become unchecked. Sometimes we need to break this cycle.

What is Dysthmia, My Experience?

One thing you have to watch out for is dysthymia, a more chronic but milder from of depression. When I was in medical school, I experienced dysthymia. I nearly went into clinical depression in the winter of my second year. It was the scariest time of my life. I did not realize what had crept up on me. I had just learned all the vegetative symptoms of depression in psychiatry class, including insomnia, lack of appetite, and slowing of activity. I had all of these and I scarcely smiled for months. I had isolated myself to study. I am a gregarious Italian and isolation and obsessive fear of not making it in medical school caused me to go downhill fast. It consumed me and I knew I had to change, or I might not make it into medical school at all.

It was the most difficult change of my life and it took me a couple of months. I had to stop isolating myself so I began interacting more with my classmates and studied with them at night. One of my kind classmates, who was admittedly more organized, took me under her wing for a few months. She called me each evening to review material and check on me and included me in her study groups. I survived that winter and the rest of medical school. I do not know what I would have done without her support.

I actually remember that on the first day of school, the librarian said to my class, "You cannot do it alone." I was naive and didn't listen. Help yourself by not over isolating in the winter. Make sure you socialize and get outside as much as possible.

TIPS FROM THE M.D.

Symptoms of Depression to Watch Out For

One in ten adults suffer from depression. Depression is the leading cause of disability in the United States for those 18 to 44.

Freud once said, "Anger turned inward is depression." I look at it in another way, obsession, this is an anger turned inward. Many of us have some burning, festering obsession, whether it is a situation at work, a relationship trauma or a life-changing event, like aging. If these obsessions go unchecked, they can bring you down.

We need to be aware of these obsessions and find ways to deal with our issues, even if we cannot immediately solve our problems. We want our problems to go away, right away, and when they don't, we worry and the trouble compounds and intensifies until the symptoms of depression may manifest. When depressed, we have a relatively constant feeling of sadness. We have trouble concentrating and our actions are slower. There are actually nine vegetative symptoms that are used to diagnosis depression.

Symptoms and Types of Anxiety

Anxiety disorders are the number one psychiatric disorder in America. Forty million Americans have some form of anxiety disorder. It is no surprise in this hectic American lifestyle we live. There are different types: Generalized Anxiety Disorder (GAD), panic attack, and post traumatic stresses disorder. Many of us have GAD and do not even know it.

Yes it is true, people are a lot of the times the source of our stress, we are social beings. However, they are also a great source of our emotional support. So do not isolate yourself in the winter or during the winter parts of your life.

It has been found that inadequate lighting, especially in the shorter days of winter, can lead to seasonal affective disorder or dysthymia. So make sure you have adequate lighting in all of your hibernation chambers at home. It is a good idea to change your furniture arrangements every so often and try to work in different rooms in your house. They have done experiments on varying the wattage on the lights in people's place of work and found that people with brighter lights are more productive.

Let's Learn From the Animals and Be Less Like Fat Bears and More Like Fastidious Penguins

So what can we learn from bears and other hibernating animals in the winter. Well, to not be like them.

It may be romantic and all, but hibernation works different in humans. Bears start out fat and lose their fat in the winter. Humans get fat when they hibernate in the winter. Maybe we can learn from the penguins and march to the gym every so often.

Before bears hibernate, they can gain forty pounds of fat a week to prepare and fatten-up before the onset of winter. There is not enough of the bear's food supply of berries (berries, great for bear anti aging too) and nuts for the bear to survive in the winter, so they must sleep to conserve energy. In hibernation, bears heart rates may drop from 55 beats per minute to about 10 beats per minute. The bear can loose fifteen to fifty percent of its body weight through the course of the winter. This is a way for the bear to survive the severe conditions of nature. We have the reverse problems. Our food resources are not a problem in the winter.

We should be more like penguins than bears. Penguins are not just the cute tuxedo birds that thrive in parts of the Antarctica that can reach 100 degrees below zero. Rockhopper penguins climb 90-foot cliffs to nest their eggs and Adelie penguins travel 3,000 miles to join breeding colonies. If penguins can do these perilous things, then you can waddle your own way to the gym at least three times a week.

By the way, penguins developed flipper boxing long before humans discovered cardio kickboxing. The sleek body of the penguin allows them to swim up to fifteen miles an hour! FYI, if we were to keep up that speed on land, it would allow us to do a four-minute mile. Don't think about hibernating all winter. Instead aspire to be like the hearty little penguin.

Winter Events in History

Although it is cold and it appears that things are slowing down, winter is certainly not a time of inactivity. January 8, 1790 witnessed the first State of the Union Address delivered by George Washington. On March 12, 1912 little girls got the chance to show up their brothers by joining the first meeting of the Girl Scouts of America. Unlike summer sports, winter sports did not have a place to gather their best athletes for decades. This all changed in January of 1924 when Chamonix, France hosted the first Official Winter Olympic Games. When you think it is too cold to be active and enjoy the season just think of those winter Olympic athletes that train to be in peak shape in the cold winter conditions.

TIPS FROM THE M.D.

Protein Requirements to Build Muscle

You want to put on muscle. Resistance training is good for the winter months. However, if you work out and do not consume enough protein, you are not going to gain muscle. So you need about 1.5 grams of protein per lean body mass to build adequate muscle. Certain health clubs have certain ways to measure your lean body mass. For example, a 130-lb. Women, her lean body mass should be between 90-100 pounds. You should consume no more than 20 grams of protein at a time. It is better to eat 5 small meals, about one meal every 3 hours.

Exercise and Calorie Burning

Did you know that if you exercise, you would burn more calories at rest than those that do not exercise? So when just sitting down, you burn more calories than your friend who did not exercise.

Research shows that you continue to burn calories after you exercise. The amount of the post-exercise elevation of energy expenditure depends mostly on the level of intensity (high, moderate or low) when you exercise and to a lesser extent, to how long you exercise. This may last about an hour afterward. Mostly the calorie burn occurs during exercise.

So what exercises provide the most calorie burn? It is important to select exercises that use large muscles of the body in continuous, rhythmic fashion and are easy to maintain at a consistent intensity.

Cycling and swimming are both non-weight-bearing exercises. Walking and jogging are weight-bearing exercises and at the same level of intensity will burn more calories. Weight bearing exercise is great for maintaining bone mass and preventing osteoporosis. But non-weight bearing exercise can be done for a longer period of time.

FEEL GOOD WINTER

I Know, It's Cold

Yes, yes, yes, it is cold, but embrace the cold and let the cold be your friend.

Watch the different patterns of snow when falling, the flurries, and the circular patterns; it's therapeutic. The wet stuff is good stuff. Every snowflake is different. Take a look sometime and see how many patterns you can find. You can do a great meditation session watching the snow from the window or get out and take a brisk walk in the quiet and still of a winter moment.

Every day when I go to my parent's house for the winter holiday, I go for a walk with my family and extended family. The Europeans do this evening walk with their family and sometimes other neighbors. When you get down in deep winter, remember the saying "In the midst of the winter, I found I had an invincible summer in me."

Winter Punch Recipe:

    1 part Activities Next to a Fireplace
    2 parts Holiday Cheer
    4 parts New Year Resolutions Leftovers
    3 parts Self-Control Around the Brownie Basket

Mix up ingredients together, blend in holiday cheer and serve next to a fireplace. Share with friend.

TIPS FOR THE WINTER WONDERLAND

53. Plan a Winter Vacation to Some Place You Have Never Been

After all the parties and excitement of the holiday season, winter can be down right depressing. Even if you can only get away for the weekend, take some time off and explore a new area. In January or February when it seems like there is no end to winter, pack your bags and get away. It will give you something to look forward when the excitement of the holiday season is behind you. It is also a good time to connect with your significant other, work colleagues, or friends. Even if you go to a cold location, getting away is the best way to avoid cabin fever.

54. Since You Will Be Home a Lot More, Spend Time De-Cluttering Your House, One Room At a Time

Forget spring-cleaning, once spring hits you will want to spend time outdoors. Why not use this time, while you are stuck indoors, to organize your home. Create a schedule of deep-cleaning and organizing projects. If you find you are going crazy at home because you are stuck inside, go to this schedule and start on a project. Put on some energizing music and start organizing.

55. Recognize the Signs of Depression and Treat Them

Depression is more than just a bout with the blues, but there are several levels of depression. The most common signs of depression are: a loss of interest in normal activities, a depressed mode including sadness, helplessness, and hopelessness, sleep disturbances, impaired concentration, changes in weight, including gaining weight or rapid weight loss, agitation, fatigue, low self-esteem, loss of interest in sex, physical pain, and thoughts of death.

If you experience these symptoms and they are severe or are affecting your work, or personal life, contact your primary care doctor. Do not let things get worse before taking steps to make them better. Depression is more common than you may realize and you shouldn't feel embarrassed asking for help.

While there is no one known cause for depression, there are several treatments for it. Talk to your doctor as soon as you experience symptoms and explore your treatment options.

56. Educate Yourself About Anxiety and Recognize the Signs

We all feel normal levels of anxiety, from a pounding heart before speaking in public or the butterflies we feel on a first date. Some levels of anxiety are good. It gears us up for challenges in life. However, if anxiety is preventing you from living how you would like to live then you may have an anxiety disorder.

The National Institute of Mental Health reports that 40 million adults are affected each year. Check with you doctor if you have anxiety which is constant, unrelenting and all consuming, or if you suffer from self-imposed isolation or emotional withdrawal. If your anxiety is interfering with normal activities, it is a good time to talk to your doctor.

How do you know that you are having an anxiety attack or panic attack?

The mental symptoms:
Apprehension, uneasiness, dread, confusion, impaired concentration or selective attention, feeling restless or on edge, self-consciousness and insecurity avoidance, irritability, behavioral problems (especially in children and adolescents), nervousness and jumpiness, fear that you are dying or going crazy, strong desire to escape.

The Physical Symptoms:
Heart palpitations or racing heartbeat, chest pain, clammy hands, stomach upset or queasiness, insomnia, frequent urination or diarrhea, shortness of breath, sweating, hot flashes or chills, dizziness, tremors, twitches, muscle tension or aches, headaches, and/or fatigue.

If you think you are suffering from anxiety, please see your doctor immediately. There are many treatments to help you.

57. Count How Many Fat Grams You Eat Each Day and Note Which Are Saturated and Which Are Not Unsaturated

Maybe you have counted your calories, but have you counted your fat grams? Pick one day, keep tract of the amount of fat grams you eat in that day. Really pay attention to the ratio of unsaturated fat (the good stuff) to saturated fat (the bad stuff). What can you do to decrease the amount of fat in your diet? How can you remove the saturated fats? Look at the list you have created and evaluate if you are eating the right kinds of food.

Fat is a flavor enhancer and is responsible for transporting that flavor to our taste buds. It also provides the creamy texture in milk, cheeses, and desserts. It is no wonder we love to eat the stuff. However, if we have too much fat, we start looking plump and feeling heavy. Try to find replacements for fat. Start by switching to good fats such as olive oil, avocados, and fish. Instead of fat, use spices to increase flavor. If you are craving that creamy texture for dessert, try low-fat alternatives like frozen yogurt, soy-based ice creams, or simply use non-fat milk when preparing your dessert.

58. Determine Your Weekly Sweet Allowance from Your Total Caloric Intake

If all you can think about is a gooey chocolate brownie then you should have one, but just one and a normal portion. The danger in depriving yourself from a craving is that you will at some point binge.

It is important to quell your sweet tooth every once in a while, but you do not need a decedent dessert every day. Winter can be a hectic time because there are so many parties and for some reason, cold weather makes everyone want to bake. Having a weekly sweet allowance will help you keep your sweet tooth from talking and your waist from growing. Learn how many calories you need in a day and reverse some for sweets. Knowing that you can have one brownie on Thursday will help you say no to cookies on Wednesday.

59. Determine Your Resistance Training Goals and Understand What Nutritional Requirements Are Needed to Maintain These Levels

No, I am not just talking to the bodybuilders. Toning-up will help increase the amount of calories your body burns when at rest to help you look even better. Resistance training increases muscle strength by forcing muscles to work against a weight or force. After a good workout, your muscles go into the anabolic phase, which lasts about 45 minutes after a strenuous workout. During this phase, muscle tissues are being rebuilt bigger than they were before, but it takes protein to do this. The amount of protein you need will vary depending your goals. Generally about 1.5 grams of protein per pound per day is recommended. Check with both your doctor and possibly a trainer about what protein amounts are correct for your body and your goals. They may also recommend supplements. The most important thing to remember is to eat a protein rich meal after your workout.

60. Plan On Taking a Walk After Dinner, Perhaps With Your Friend(s) Or Family

Unless you live in a big city, you probably don't walk enough. The next time you have dinner with a friend suggest a post-dinner stroll. Finish your conversation while walking, instead of over dessert. Think of the Europeans who stroll down the street together, enjoying each other's company.

If you eat at home, walk around your block and see what new things you can notice. If a park is nearby, stroll through the park in the early evening. If you go out to a restaurant, walk around that neighborhood and take a look at the shops or anything else the neighborhood has to offer. And if it is just too plain cold, stroll around an indoor mall and window shop.

61. Pick Up Isokinetic Bands To Use In The Hotel Room or at Home

If we are not stuck at home, we are often traveling during the winter months. From long days, to interrupted sleep patterns, to heavy meals, traveling can leave you tired and drained. What's worse is that you skip your regular workout routine and have little to no activity.

Isokinetic bands are a great way to exercise in the privacy of your hotel room. They are elastic resistance bands with handles on each end. They are inexpensive and small enough to pack. Check out the website for recommended isokinetic exercises you can do anywhere.

What exactly is an isokinetic band? An isokinetic band is a rubber tube that you can stretch to work out. You can put these in your suitcase and pull them out when you are in your hotel room to exercise. Get that valuable resistance training in at home, in your hotel room, or at the in-laws house.

62. Try Out One Indoor Sport With a Friend (Tennis, Basketball, Swimming, Indoor Jogging)

I know it is more challenging to stay active in the winter in some climates. Even in the most temperate location, it may be colder or raining. However, there are indoor golf driving ranges and hitting golf balls can be a great way to get out any aggression you are feeling while exercising some muscle groups. Tennis, racquetball and basketball can all be played indoors. Gyms, and occasionally recreation centers, have indoor pools. Try going for a mid-winter swim to stay in shape. For those of you who are more daring, many cities have an indoor trapeze. Try something new and keep your eye out for sports and activities that can be done indoors when weather outside is less permitting.

63. Develop a Morning and Evening Stretching Program

This should be an easy one because you can do this in front of your television and it should only take about fifteen minutes each morning and each evening. Stretching your body in the morning is a great way to loosen and invigorate your muscles. Proper stretching will increase your blood flow and help you wake up faster. Evening stretches should calm your body and work out any kinks you have developed during the day. Stretching is a great way to relax yourself before going to bed.

Ask a trainer at your gym for some recommended stretches or find a fifteen-minute yoga video. There are several morning/evening stretching videos available as well. Just a few dedicated moments each day will have you feeling good, and you should start sleeping better.

64. Get at Least One Personal Training Session

I know, it would be so much easier to get in shape if you could get out of your bed, have a trainer come to your house and force you to work out at an optimum level every day. Perhaps a personal chef to prepare delicious, yet healthy meals would help too. While most of us are unable to swing all that, we usually can afford at least one or two professional training sessions.

Find personal trainer that is ACE certified and has a good knowledge of nutrition. You can find potential trainers at a gym, a private training studio, or simply independent trainers who advertise in local magazines or online.

Trainers are so valuable because they can assess where you are at in relation to your goals. Trainers will set-up a plan for you to reach your goals, teach you proper form and technique, and provide encouragement. Your fist appointment should be an evaluation where your measurements, weight, and fat percentage are taken. No, it's not painful and you will appreciate these initial values when you look back later.

The more sessions you can do, the better. Even it you can only do one or two you will benefit greatly from meeting with a professional.

65. Recognize the Early Symptoms of a Cold and Address Them Immediately

You know that feeling. You try to ignore it, but there was something different about that last sneeze and your throat is starting to tickle. You are "coming down with something." This is the time to take care of yourself and treat the cold now. So take it easy and do the bare minimum to get through your obligations during the day. You can perhaps prevent a full-blown cold from developing. Make sure you are properly hydrated with fluids and above everything else, rest! Taking a few extra hours to let your body rest now may prevent the cold from developing and knocking you out for days.

Early symptoms of a cold include sneezing and runny nose, sore throat, watering eyes, headache, and general malaise. Most symptoms appear about two days after you have been infected. While there is no cure to the common cold, you can certainly decrease the symptoms and the length of your cold by maintaining proper nutrition, resting, and staying hydrated.

66. Avoid Eating When Bored, Learn To Recognize Hunger

Boredom eating is very common and even more dangerous in the winter when we spend more time indoors around sweets and other treats. Check yourself before you start eating. Are you really hungry or are you bored? Emotionally eating, or satisfying an impulse craving?

True hunger feels like a mild gnawing sensation in your stomach. While I would never suggest that you wait until you are famished, make sure you are really hungry before you eat. If you find yourself heading for a snack, ask yourself, "How hungry am I?" Try drinking a glass of water first or snacking on carrots, celery or fruit. When you are truly hungry, all foods taste good, not just the fattening ones. If the carrots, celery or fruit doesn't sound good to you, then were you really hungry in the first place? Also, keep in mind that is takes about twenty minutes for your brain to register a full feeling. So, when you do eat, slow down, chew thoroughly and enjoy each bite. Take a few breaks to contribute to a conversation or put your fork down for a moment. Stop eating when you feel satisfied, not when you feel painfully full.

67. Take Care of Your Kisser

The most important thing you can do for you lips is to drink enough water. To keep your lips soft and supple, use a lip balm each night that is fortified with vitamins. Your lips can burn in the sunlight too and it can be quite painful, so make sure your balm has an SPF in it as well.

Another way to avoid chapped lips is to stop licking them. Licking your lips will dry them out.

Ladies, put a basecoat of a lip balm on prior to applying you lipstick. If you do happen to have chapped lips, then avoid lipsticks for a while, they can really dry out your lips.

Gentlemen, you need to moisture your lips too. If you hate having a balm on during the day, try applying it at night.

68. Learn How To Reduce Fat From Steaks and Chicken

Sometimes you just crave meat and there is no denying it.

If it is steak you are craving then enjoy it. It is ok to have a steak every once in a while. When the time comes to enjoy a delicious cut of meat, do the following: choose a lean cut of beef like a filet or NY strip, avoid rib eyes and other fatty cuts, and when possible, trim away all of the visible fat.

If you are hankering for some chicken, then remove the skin and cut off the visible pieces of fat. There is absolutely no redeeming value to the skin. Opt for preparation methods that do not add fat, like baking, boiling or grilling. If you need to add flavor, try various seasonings or fat-free marinades. You do not need to deep fry chicken to enjoy it. Try a sauté or stir-fry, but if you use any oil, make it olive oil.

69. Eat Fish That Is Rich In Omega-3 Fatty Acids

What is the deal with omega-3 fatty acids? Omega-3 fatty acids are essential acids that cannot be manufactured by our bodies. These essential fatty acids must come from our diets. Even though we can make them, omega-3's play several valuable rolls in the human body. A crucial role is in brain function and normal growth and development. They have been shown to reduce inflammation and prevent chronic disease, such as heart disease and arthritis. Omega-3's are important for cognitive and behavioral function. Cultures that have diets high in omega-3 fatty acids are some of the healthiest people in the world. Just take a look at the Mediterranean diet.

Increase the amount of omega-3 fatty acids your consuming by eating salmon, trout, and herring. Try to eat fish at least twice a week.

70. Identify the Different Physical Needs Between You and Your Significant Other

If you are both stuck inside your home, take this time to really connect with one another. Turn off the television and spend time together without distractions. Talk about the physical needs you both have and find ways to make time for each other and address those most intimate needs. It is important to keep your romantic relationship exciting and fulfilling. If you have needs that your partner is not meeting then talk about it. Don't forget to give praise where praise is warranted. The goal is to have a comfortable, open discussion, which will help you connect better with your partner in the bedroom and in life as well.

71. Have Adequate Lighting In Every Room of Your House

Millions of people suffer from Seasonal Affective Disorder (SAD) each year. Although people living in colder areas with less daylight are more affected, no one is exempt. Yes, even people in sunny Southern California and Florida can suffer from the winter blues. Filling your house with adequate lighting can ease the severity of SAD. There are also light boxes available online that use bright blue lights to boost your mood. In severe cases doctors can prescribe mood elevators.

72. At Parties, Yes, Those Crazy Holiday Parties..., Drink Alcohol in Moderation

Everyone has a good holiday story or two, usually from office holiday parties when so-and-so from accounting really cut loose. Don't be one of those stories. You could do without the humiliation, the hangover, and the calories. The recommended amount is one drink for women and two drinks for men. Sorry ladies, it is just because you weigh less. If you feel like you need a drink in your hand, try this: start with water and get yourself hydrated first, tell the drink pusher that you will have a drink in a moment, when everyone is moving onto round two, have one drink and sip it. Stick with wine or drinks with soda water. Most of those fancy cocktails have almost as many calories as a full meal. When you are done with your first drink, return to water for the next round, sip, repeat (for men).

73. Take a Yoga Class

If you have not tried one of the oldest forms of exercise and mental relaxation, the time has come for you to stretch out your yoga mat and get busy. Often, people who have never done yoga think that you must be flexible before starting or that you may have to keep up with others during a class. The truth is, yoga has little to do with your initial flexibility. Yoga is about the breath. You will learn how to connect your body to your mind and just breathe. Meanwhile, your flexibility will naturally increase.

Yoga has so many health benefits, including physiological, psychological and biochemical. Doing yoga regular can decrease your blood pressure, increase your energy level, decrease any pain, elevate your mood and concentration, decrease anxiety and depression, while decreasing your total cholesterol and bringing about favorable body reaction.

Perhaps you already have a penchant for yoga, but you don't want to go full force and join a yoga studio. Instead, take just one class at a time. You don't even need to buy expensive gear. Most studios and even gyms provide yoga mats.

Little known fact: most yoga studios will let you try your first class for free.

74. Try Tofu, Turkey, Tuna or Veggie Burgers

I'm not forcing you to give up meat, but if you are going to eat healthier and stay within your recommended daily calorie intake, it is good to have a few low calorie, low-fat alternatives. Tofu has all sorts of applications many don't even know about. For example, the extra-firm style is terrific for those looking for a more meat-like bite. Slice it up and add to a salad. Tofu also great in stir-fry, baked dishes, and burgers.

Turkey is a great source of lean meat. It is filling and good for you. Roast a turkey breast and slice for meals or, keep the leftovers for sandwiches. Replace your fattening ground beef with lower fat ground turkey.

Tuna is also a fantastic source of lean protein. Buy the water packed version instead of the tuna packed in oil. Add tuna to a hearty salad or stir-in with pasta – how European of you! If you want to make a tuna salad, use less mayo or choose a light/fat-free version. Use seasonings to add flavor and enjoy with a few whole-wheat crackers.

A good veggie burger can also be quite tasty. Sometimes you will need to try a few brands before finding one that suites your tastes. You should also be mindful of fat and calories in veggie burgers. Read labels because some veggie burgers use cheese to add flavor and fat, not good.

75. Order In Healthy Takeout and Play a Board Game. This Will Engage Your Friends More Than Watching Television Shows or Movies

The television is out this year and board games are in. These new games are not the games of our childhood. Monopoly is a classic, but have you tried Battle of the Sexes, Cranium, and Balderdash? Play games that are interactive. Take the time to laugh with your friends, while you challenge each other to sudden death in Cranium.

Perhaps all you have is a deck of cards-then play five-card draw, Texas hold'em or gin rummy. This is a great way to be interactive and learn more about your friends. Winter is the worst time for seasonal affective disorder, especially in February and March. Remember, the house always wins when you beat cabin fever.

76. Learn the Difference Between Bronchitis and Pneumonia

Many of my patients come in and are concerned that they may have pneumonia or a serious infection in their lungs. Pneumonia is an infection of the lungs proper when the lungs fill-up with the cells that fight infection. If a virus causes the pneumonia, then it is viral pneumonia and if bacteria cause the infection, then it is a bacterial pneumonia. The main symptoms are shortness of breath, cough, fever, sputum production and sharp chest pain when you breathe. Bronchitis like the name implies is an "itis" or infection of the central bronchial tubes, and can be viral or bacterial. Bronchitis may have some of the same symptoms, but may not be associated with shortness of breath. Your doctor can distinguish between the breath sounds of the two when they listen to your lungs. Bacterial pneumonia and bronchitis, and some viral pneumonias, need to be treated with antibiotics. Pneumonia can be in fact life threatening in the elderly.

77. Bundle Up and Take a Winter Walk Saturday or Sunday morning

This can really clear your mind. The crisp, cool air in the still of a winter morning can be a form of meditation. Winter skies are some of the most clear and most beautiful. Make your walk a progressive walk, perhaps with your neighbors or a friend. Go from house-to-house, either serving small appetizers or warm drinks for a twist of something different.

On a clear winter night, carry a blanket and sit outside and stargaze with your friends.

This will prevent you from becoming one of those hibernating bears.

78. Roll Up Your Sleeves and Do an Act of Charity

Extend the spirit and give beyond your family and friends. There are so many opportunities to help people who are less privileged. Spend time getting to know the people in your community face-to-face, who need your donation and your support. Feel good about giving and getting in touch with your community.

We all have different gifts to offer that extend beyond volunteering in a soup kitchen. Check out volunteermatch.com to find a charity or someone in need near you. Helping others is a great way to give back and feel good about yourself.

WINTER TIPS PLANNER

Choose your two tips per week and place them under the heading, below called Tip #.

Put a line through each chosen tip after you have mastered it.

	Date	Tip #
Week 1	_____	_____
Week 2	_____	_____
Week 3	_____	_____
Week 4	_____	_____
Week 5	_____	_____
Week 6	_____	_____
Week 7	_____	_____
Week 8	_____	_____
Week 9	_____	_____
Week 10	_____	_____
Week 11	_____	_____
Week 12	_____	_____
Week 13	_____	_____

FEEL GOOD SUMMER TRACKER

Ideal Body Weight and Deviance +/- from the Ideal

Ideal Body Weight _____

December 21 _____
January weight *(within the 1st week)* _____
February weight *(within the 1st week)* _____
March weight *(within the 1st week)* _____

Total Calorie Intake Maintenance, Weight Loss, to Build Muscle
(your goals may change throughout the year, see www.feelgoodhealthnow.com)

Total Daily Calorie/Fat Gram/
    Protein Gram Intake for Maintenance _____
Total Daily Calorie/Fat Gram/
    Protein Gram Intake for Weight Loss _____
Total Daily Calorie/Fat Gram/
    Protein Intake to Build Muscle _____

Target Heart Rate for Aerobic Exercise
(see www.feelgoodhealthnow.com)

Moderate Intensity THR _____
High Intensity THR _____

FEEL GOOD WINTER

Stressors: *(work, family, personal, financial or environmental)*
_____
_____
_____

Plan to cope with above stressors: _____
_____
_____
_____

Average Feel Good Score (1 to 10)
("1" is Completely Lousy and "10" is Blissful)

December 21   _____
January *(within the 1st week)* Date/Score   _____
February *(within the 1st week)* Date/Score   _____
March *(within the 1st week)* Date/Score   _____

Tips or life changes that increased your feel good score:
_____
_____
_____
_____
_____
_____
_____

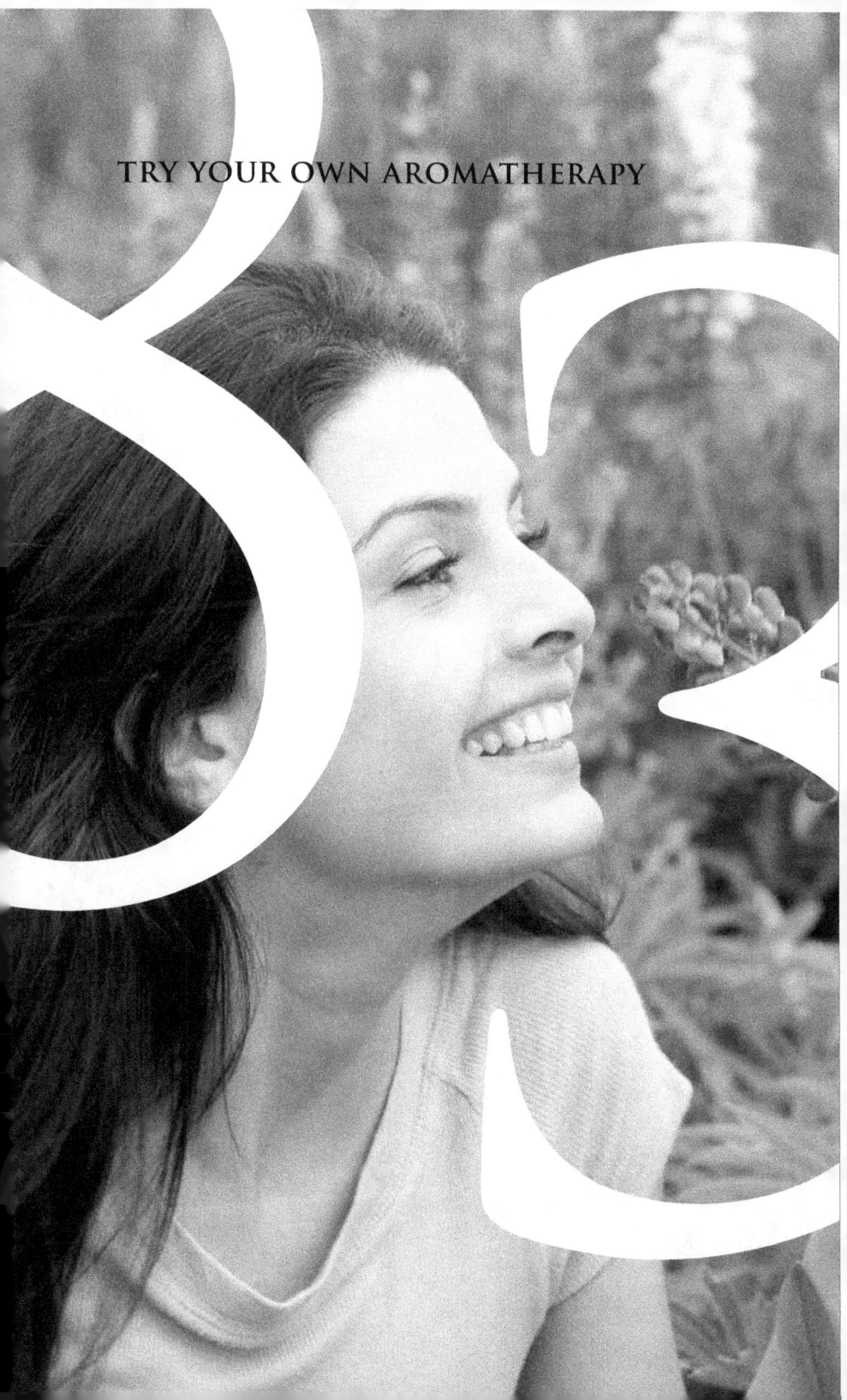

TRY YOUR OWN AROMATHERAPY

FEEL GOOD SPRING

SPRING

"Spring is nature's way of saying, "Let's party"
— Robin Williams

GOALS FOR SPRING

Knockout Stress:
Learn to identify stressors in your life and then combat these stresses by implementing basic, stress management techniques. Over time, implement a daily and then a weekly plan to manage work and home stress.

Make Your Calories Count:
Count your calories and learn to eliminate empty calories, replacing them with nutrient-rich, delicious foods.

Electrify Your Body:
Increase your energy levels by participating in moderate or vigorous exercise and learning the concept of target heart rates.

Time To Let Your Skin Shine:
Learn to take care of the external part of your body: your face, hair and skin. Take steps to keep it looking good and to prevent cancer.

FEEL GOOD SPRING

Winter slowly disappears, the weather gradually gets warmer and we know that spring is finally here. Spring is a time to both take command of your stresses and to take time to smell the roses. I will outline several steps to bring your stress level down and really enjoy this season and all the seasons in your future, which will be longer once you get a handle on your stress. So you ask, "How do we smell the roses?" We smell them with our nose of course, but more importantly, with an attitude of appreciation.

When I think of spring, the first memories that come back to me are the great smells of the season. What are pleasing smells to you? Think back, when you where playing outside during grade school - what smells do you remember?

Did you live near a forest and smell oak trees and earth? Did you have a big yard with fruit trees and planted flowers or lilac bushes? Did you live in the city and smell the flowers in the parks or the smell of springtime in the city.

TIPS FROM THE M.D.

The Nose and Its Vital Functions

The nose is no joke.
The nose has 3 functions; to moisten air, filter it as we breathe, and to facilitate smell.

The truth is smell doesn't get the credit it deserves. Our sense of smell allows us to enjoy the scent of fresh flowers, ocean breezes, and even enhances the taste of our foods. However, the sense of smell plays an even more important roll. Our sense of smell can save our lives. If we smell smoke from a fire, we know to stay away, or if we smell rotten food we know not to eat it. Ever hear that pregnant women have a heightened sense of smell? Their sense of smell becomes more discerning to protect their unborn baby.

How do we smell?
There are two olfactory membranes, smelling surfaces, under the bridge of our noses that are about as big as a postage stamp. As we breathe in the vapors are dissolved and the olfactory nerve, the smelling nerve, converts those smells into electrical signals. Generally, signals going to the brain have to travel throughout the body to reach the brain. However, the smelling nerve goes straight back to the part of the brain that stores memory and feelings without any detours to the cerebral cortex. This is why there is a strong memory connection with the sense of smell.

FEEL GOOD SPRING

Smells Like Springtime

My favorite smell memories from spring come from when I was in high school. I used to run along a road next to a river and would often smell the scent of the birch trees. When I pass by a birch tree now, the memory from those runs comes flooding back. The smell of those trees makes me feel happy and young again.

Smells are powerful memory triggers and the relationship between smell and memory has been the subject of many studies.

In fact, in the 1930's, Edward Bach came up with the Bach Flower remedies. He left his London medical practice to study flower essences, he came up with 38 flower essences that each defined an aspect of human nature. These extracts were used to treat anxiety and depression. When you see all the blossoms and new flowers that come out in spring, stop and enjoy the smell, you never know how much they may be relaxing you subconsciously.

Although spring can be exciting and revitalizing, it can also be a time of uncertainty. The weather is uncertain. We don't know when spring will finally start or if it will rain for another week. I have spent many Memorial Day picnics uncertain if we should start the grill, or if the rain would prevent an outdoor gathering. We are also uncertain just how bad the winter has worn on our body and minds. The changing of the weather and the transition from the harshness of winter to a lighter spring can bring about other changes in our lives. We have to shed old habits and sometimes relationships change.

Take Control of Your Stress

So how do we handle this uncertainty and make sure we can feel better about the stresses in our lives?

Stress is nebulous uncertainty. We must first get a hold of stress, pinpointing its causes and start dealing with them. Stress comes from different parts of our lives. We can have environmental stress, work, family, and significant other stress. Then, there is financial stress, which is a category unto itself.

There is a way to manage and deal with these stresses. The first step is to go through certain exercises and rate our level of stress from one to ten. We should keep a daily stress diary of all our stresses.

We then need to access the adequacy of our support system. There are three types of support: informational, financial and emotional. To better fight stress, we need an emotional back up. We need to call on our support system, a friend who is honest, sincere and may have some wisdom and insight into the particular problem that is getting under your skin.

Spring is a great time to start implementing a stress management system. This season I will discuss tips on how to assess your support system and how to utilize it best. But remember, any good relationship is give and take; so be prepared to help them out in their time of need. We will discuss how to deal with your stresses cognitively, with relaxation techniques, exercise and nutrition for stress.

I will arm you with other stress reduction techniques, such as deep breathing, progressive muscular relaxation and therapeutic laughter. I will give you tips that help you de-stress during your workday and lifestyle tips that will help you better cope with stress.

Spring is also a time to take inventory of your body and mind, of where you want to go and where you have been.

Now that winter is over, let's take time to check our bodies closely and think about what might be going on undetected and unseen.

The Unforeseen Cancer

Quiz time, what do gasoline, nitrates, asbestos and smoking having in common? Yes, you guessed it, these are all carcinogens. How does cancer start? It starts form a mutation, an alteration of one cell. Yes – one cell is all it takes. This one bad apple may multiply for years before we discover it.

This season we will discuss these different carcinogens in our environment and how to limit them so they do not progress to cancer. About half a million people die of cancer every year and one-third of these cancers can be prevented by better diet and exercise.

So, early detection is important to stop this one cell before it divides and gets to the point where it cannot be stopped. We will discuss the prevention guidelines for breast, prostate, and skin cancers. I will recommend certain supplements to take that have some promise in stopping cancer.

We all have a perception of our body, but do we really understand our physical make-up. Next time you go to a massage therapist, and I do recommend this often, have them give you an anatomy lesson.

It is time to get organized from head-to-toe for prevention.

To keep you on track, here are some of the things you should have in a morning and evening ritual. In the morning, you should think about teeth, skin, and sunscreen. In the evening you should think about replenishing the moisture your skin has lost throughout the day. But don't forget to brush. Brushing your teeth is important in the evening, so bacteria does not rest on your teeth when you are sleeping.

Everyone wants to improve his or her energy level. Do you know you can eat to feel better and improve you energy level? If time permits, it is best to have five small meals a day, eating a smaller amount of food each time. In the hospital, I do a calorie count of my patients that I suspect are not getting enough calories a day, however, most Americans have the opposite problem. It is a good idea to assess the total calories a day you are consuming. Choose one day and do a calorie count. Every little bite counts and you may be surprised by how many calories you are really consuming in a day.

Basically, most of the food you put in your frig should be of high nutritional content. Eating the right foods will make you feel better. Try it for a day. Eat right and test your feel good index on a scale from 1 to 10 – "1" being lousy and "10" being absolutely blissful. Note how you feel throughout the day and then note how much easier it is to wake up and how great you feel the next day.

In spring, we start to get anxious about the impending swimsuit season. After months of a sedentary life style, we jump reluctantly into workout mode. We must first assess our aerobic capabilities and then get started. How does this relate to feeling good? Quite frankly, aerobic exercise is addictive. You can seriously get a feeling of elation with aerobic exercise. Ever hear of a runner's high? If that doesn't motivate you, remember that every hour that you spend exercising will increase you life by three hours, not to mention improve the overall quality.

So let's assess how in or out of shape we are. If you are not in shape, don't worry, you are not alone. 86% of Americans are out of shape. Certain individuals may not have the capacity to do exercise at more intense levels, but most people do. You are in acceptable shape if you can sustain moderate intensity exercise for at least 20 minutes at a time.

How much should you be exercising? Well the American Heart Association recommends exercising three times a week for at least thirty minutes. Do you know there are 336 thirty-minute blocks in a week? If you calculate for a 40-hour workweek, time for adequate sleep (about fifty-six hours), grooming, meals and transportation time, you still have left over 126 thirty-minute blocks to get in three thirty-minute blocks of exercise. No more excuses.

I recommend that you make workout time a feel good time. Buy functional workout clothes that are flattering and make you feel good. When you workout, get into the zone. You should focus on two things, proper form and relaxing without being lazy. Just relax and do not think of that passive aggressive boss or that deadline tomorrow, but instead, think of that upcoming vacation or how great you will look in your new, toned body.

Quiz time again. How much exercise do you do in a day? How much walking do you do during the course of a whole day? Do you use the elevator, even it you only have to go up one or two floors? You know who you are, and you know what to do. Follow the spring tips and increase the amount of exercise you get in a day.

I encourage you to learn how to use an exercise ball, free weights, or resistance bands. You need to have a routine of exercises you can do at home, in your bedroom or in front of the TV. I know a lot of you spend time in front of the TV relaxing, so why don't you try to get in one of those 30-minute workouts during your show. Perhaps not your favorite shows, when you are less likely to focus on the workout fully.

TIPS FROM THE M.D.

Target Heart Rates

Just what are target heart rates? You may have heard this buzzword before. Target heart rates define what target you should try to get your heart rate up to for the full psychological and cardiopulmonary benefit of aerobic exercise. It is how fast your heart should be beating at the end of your workout to achieve the best benefit for your heart, lungs and circulatory system. Aerobic exercise has proven to be of benefit in controlling stress and treating anxiety and depression. You can do exercise at a moderate intensity or a high intensity. The most body and mind benefits occur when you do high intensity work out.

Here is how we calculate Target Heart Rates (THR).

THR for moderate intensity exercise:

Subtract your age from 220. Once you find that number, multiply it by 0.625.

(220 – your age) X 0.625

Example – If you are 20 and you want to do a moderate intensity work out, you would take 220 and subtract 20 from it, resulting in 200. You would then multiply 200 by 0.625 and get 125

(220 – 20) x 0.625 = 125 beats per minute

THR for high intensity workout
(220 – your age) X 0.85

If you are 20 and want to make sure you are getting a high intensity workout you would subtract 20 from 220 and get 200. You would then multiply 200 by 0.85 and get 170

(220 – 20) x 0.85 = 170 beats per minute

How To Take Your Pulse

Starting with your hand palm side up, take you index finger and middle finger and slide them down your thumb to your radial pulse area on your wrist. Find your pulse by placing your two fingers slightly more to your thumb side from the middle of your wrist. Pause for a moment and give yourself time to feel for it. Once you find your pulse, count the pulsations for 6 seconds, and then multiply the number by 10. This is your pulse or heart rate. Try this while sitting in a quiet room the first time.

Our normal resting pulse is 60 to 100. When you want to calculate your target heart rate, you should check your pulse at the end of the workout to see if you have achieved this goal.

Recipe For Spring Cocktail:

- 1 part Stress-Free Decompression
- 2 parts Emotional and Mental Balance
- 4 parts Energy Infused Enthusiasm
- 2 parts New Goals and Knowledge

Mix ingredients together, removing any apprehension that may appear. Can be served hot or cold.

your heart rate up to for the full psychological and cardiopulmonary benefit of aerobic exercise. It is how fast your heart should be beating at the end of your workout to achieve the best benefit for your heart, lungs and circulatory system. Aerobic exercise has proven to be of benefit in controlling stress and treating anxiety and depression. You can do exercise at a moderate intensity or a high intensity. The most body and mind benefits occur when you do high intensity work out.

Here is how we calculate Target Heart Rates (THR).

THR for moderate intensity exercise:

Subtract your age from 220. Once you find that number, multiply it by 0.625.

(220 − your age) X 0.625

Example − If you are 20 and you want to do a moderate intensity work out, you would take 220 and subtract 20 from it, resulting in 200. You would then multiply 200 by 0.625 and get 125

(220 − 20) x 0.625 = 125 beats per minute

THR for high intensity workout
(220 − your age) X 0.85

If you are 20 and want to make sure you are getting a high intensity workout you would subtract 20 from 220 and get 200. You would then multiply 200 by 0.85 and get 170

(220 − 20) x 0.85 = 170 beats per minute

How To Take Your Pulse

Starting with your hand palm side up, take you index finger and middle finger and slide them down your thumb to your radial pulse area on your wrist. Find your pulse by placing your two fingers slightly more to your thumb side from the middle of your wrist. Pause for a moment and give yourself time to feel for it. Once you find your pulse, count the pulsations for 6 seconds, and then multiply the number by 10. This is your pulse or heart rate. Try this while sitting in a quiet room the first time.

Our normal resting pulse is 60 to 100. When you want to calculate your target heart rate, you should check your pulse at the end of the workout to see if you have achieved this goal.

Recipe For Spring Cocktail:

- 1 part Stress-Free Decompression
- 2 parts Emotional and Mental Balance
- 4 parts Energy Infused Enthusiasm
- 2 parts New Goals and Knowledge

Mix ingredients together, removing any apprehension that may appear. Can be served hot or cold.

Spring Moments In History

April was also the month that the first, certified organic restaurant was opened. An authentic, organic restaurant means that 95% or more of everything that you eat in the restaurant has been produced by certified, organic growers and farmers.

Give them bread, no beer. On May 8, 1842, Emil Christian, the father of the beer industry was born. Beers lovers, take praise, the Danish botanist revolutionized the beer industry, by proving that there were different species of yeast. He refused to patent the method, and made it available and free to brewers everywhere. Let's have a drink to this man for beer lovers everywhere…Hey, I said one drink!

Chicken or Chicken. On May 15, 1930, Mrs. Ellen Church, a registered nurse, became the world's first airline stewardess or today, flight attendant. The United flight flew 11 passengers from San Francisco to Cheyenne, Wyoming. Ellen served them chicken, fruit salad and rolls.

SPRING INTO ACTION TIPS

79. Make Your Time to Workout More Efficient

Start by setting out your clothes the night before you workout. This will get you focused first thing in the morning. Establish a workout routine. Do you do free weights on Mondays or Fridays and yoga on Tuesdays and Thursdays? Have a plan for your workout. This way you won't waste time trying to decide which exercises to do. There is also a better chance that you will complete a full workout. You may want to consult a personal trainer. Often trainers are happy to meet with you a few times to develop a schedule and to show you how to properly do the exercises.

80. Pinpoint Your Major Stresses in Your Work Life

What are your work stresses? Is it a person or a situation? Do you have a great deal of stress with your getting to work or dealing with the weather?

Record your daily stresses and rate them. Try to understand why these particular stresses bother you.

Sometimes simply getting out of the office for 10 to 20 min will help so get some exercise and get out of the office and take a walk by yourself or with a co-worker or neighbor.

TIPS FOR THE M.D.

The Proper Amount of Sleep

We need energy to fight stress. We need the right amount of sleep to get the energy every day to fight anxiety and stress. The proper amount of sleep varies from individual to individual. It ranges from about 6.5 to 9 hours. Many Americans are not getting enough sleep. If you are catching up on the weekends or on vacation, then you are not getting enough sleep. Basically, you should have that refreshed feeling every morning when you wake up not just after the catch up sleep. Americans are sleeping 1 to 1.5 hours less than they did from the early part of the 20th century. Maybe there is something to people who do get enough sleep; Albert Einstein got 10 hours of sleep.

81. Go On Your Own Out-of-the-Ordinary Field Trip – A Museum, Community Center or Spa

Get out there and do something different. If you haven't been to the traditional museums in a while, spend an afternoon in an art, history or science museums. If you have been there and done that, find unusual museums. Does your city have a surfing museum, Beatle memorabilia, or all things blue museum? Find something fun that will educate you and make you laugh. Check out some of the various community or cultural centers in your city. Or spend the day at a spa relaxing and pampering yourself.

82. Make Sure You Incorporate Foods Rich in Antioxidant Content

Antioxidant rich foods will help prevent cancer and heart disease, reduce blood pressure, and slow the effects of aging. What are the top antioxidant rich foods? The top antioxidant foods are berries, broccoli, tomatoes, red grapes and garlic. What drink is rich in antioxidants? The world's most popular drink tea. Either black or green teas are both high in antioxidant levels. The grains in whole grain cereal are rich in Vitamin E, a potent antioxidant.

83. Try Your Own Aromatherapy

Literally smell the roses. Aromatherapy is a practice that uses plant oils and essential oils for psychological and physical well being. These are natural oils and not artificial fragrance oils. The naturally occurring chemicals offer many benefits if they are smelled or if the oils are rubbed directly on the skin. Some oils may need special handling so be sure to consult the website to find out information. Just finding feel good smells around your house may also lift your mood. Try your own aromatherapy by going to an arboretum or a park and ask one of the park guides to help you smell roses and other Spring flowers that have pleasing smells. Also, find a bath soap that invigorates your day or change your home fragrance to a scent that reflects spring.

84. Start or Join a Laughter Group

How many times a day do you laugh? Do you know we laugh about 100 times more as a child? Groups get together to laugh to learn how to laugh and perhaps do an exercise when they laugh. The laughter leader actually teaches people physically how to laugh. Laughter is a powerful stress reliever and It Is said two hours of laughing is equivalent to 8 hours of restful sleep.

People meet for laughter yoga. Yes, that is right, laughter yoga – a blend of yogic deep breathing, stretching and simulated laughter exercises.

85. Eat More Unsaturated and Polyunsaturated Fats and Less Saturated and Trans Fats

Unsaturated, monounsaturated, Trans fats, hydrogenated, poly – what? With all the terms out there it is easy to get confused and even harder to figure out what to eat. These terms refer to chemical processes or to chemical structure composition, but let's leave the chemistry to the chemist. To explain it in simpler terms:

Trans Fatty Acids:
Trans fats, also called hydrogenated fats are fake fats (well, they occur naturally in small amounts in meats). These fats were created by scientists for the packaged food industry and are extremely unhealthy. In fact many restaurants and even cities have banned them. Why were they created? Well, because many fats are liquid at room temperature, like olive oil for example. But what if you want your

chocolate bar to travel from the candy factory to the grocery store to the consumer and never melt… and you want to do it cheaply? You would perform a chemical process on the fat called hydrogenation. This process chemically alters the fat so that it stays solid at room temperature. Yum! These fats are terrible for you and should be completely avoided.

Saturated Fat:
These are not the best for you but can be enjoyed in small amounts. Saturated fats include meat, animal fats, butter, creams, and cheeses. These foods are the main cause of dietary cholesterol. Arguably better for you than Trans fats, saturated fat should be consumed in moderation.

Unsaturated Fat:
Unsaturated fats are the best fats for you. These are the healthy fats that lower over all blood cholesterol. These fats include fish, nuts, seeds, and many oils. As an added benefit many unsaturated fats contain omega-3-fatty acids. More "good for you" stuff.

86. Understand the General Aspects of the Food Guide Pyramid

In 2005, The American Dietetic Association updated the pyramid now is a food and exercise pyramid. The food has 6 parts. The first group is for grains. Remember to have at least half of our grains whole grains. The nest group is for vegetables. Remember to eat dark green and orange veggies. Third is the fruit group, fresh frozen, canned or dried. Forth, milk products, try low fat or fat free Fifth, meat and beans,

Choose lean meats and poultry, fish at least twice a week, nuts and seeds Finally, the last food group is oils, choose monounsaturated and poly-unsaturated oils. The ADA has steps on the pyramid to remind us to be active every day. Yes, every day is best.

Go to mypyrimid.gov to find out your total caloric intake and how much of each food group you should have.

87. Get and Use an Exercise Ball

An exercise ball is a great tool because they are so versatile and quite inexpensive. From abdominal work, to lower backstretches to full bodywork, there are endless strength training exercises that can be done on an exercise ball. Have a trainer at your gym show to how to use an exercise ball or pickup a video trainer. Online stores have hundreds, but try looking in a video or sports store first. Exercise balls can be deflated and are easy to store. It is a great accompaniment to your home exercise equipment.

88. Learn How to Apply Your Target Heart Rates When You Use a Treadmill or Any Exercise

If you are not hitting your target heart rate then you are not getting the most from your workouts. To make sure you are hitting your target heart rate and to learn what exercising at this level feels like – try it out on a treadmill as you walk or jog. Even if you have to go to a store that sells treadmills or get a one-day pass to a friend's gym, try it out! To calculate your target heart rates see the opening of this section.

89. Limit or Avoid These Carcinogens: Benzene (an additive in gasoline), Lead, Asbestos, Processed Meats and Yes, The Biggy, Smoking

Carcinogens are agents know to cause cancer. Many of the carcinogens listed above probably did not surprise you, but what about lunchmeat? Yes, lunchmeat is a carcinogen. Overly processed and packed with chemicals like nitric oxide, lunchmeat has been linked to pancreatic cancer and other health issues. Searching for something to put in your sandwich? Try roasting or baking turkey or chicken breast on the weekend and slicing it for sandwiches and salads during the week.

If you are still smoking it is time to stop. Period.

90. Buy Some Snazzy New Workout Clothes

Buying new clothes can be a great motivating factor for getting you to workout, run outdoors, or hit the gym. If you look good and feel good in your new workout duds, you will want to go to the gym more. Of course if you are getting a really great workout then you are going to sweat so don't be too concerned with how you look.

New gear can motivate you too as well and teach you something new. Use a heart monitor to make sure you are hitting your target heart rate or buy an ipod. For even more motivation try loading your ipod with your favorite fast past songs. Get out there are strut your stuff.

91. Rate Your Stress Score Using a Stress Scale

Take a stress diary. Pick one weekday and one weekend day and take note of all the stresses that occur in a day. Take note of every noise, the severe weather, the traffic, the rude store clerk, waiting in line, the friend who hung up on you because you said you were going to be late arriving at the gym. Rank these stresses from 1 to 10. 1 being the small stuff that you should perhaps let go and 10 being the worst kind of stress you could imagine. We all have stress, it is unavoidable, but it is important how we take it in, interpret it and how we react to it. We should take note of the belief that we attach to it – try not to have 2 life changing events at the same time

What scale are you using?

92. Assess Your Support System – Work, Friends, and Family

None of us is fully strong mentally through the whole year. We need a robust support system that can come to our aid when we are stressed in any one aspect of our life. Do you have enough friends either at work or understand the dynamics you face at work? Sometimes, certain wise friends know you and the situation you're facing at work that they can prevent problems form occurring altogether or limit the damage. Do you have someone who has some idea about your personal life to advise you? In general, you want to choose friends who are emotionally stable, honest and sincere to help you.

93. Do a One-Day Calorie Count and Compare Your Number to Your Caloric Needs for the Day

This can be extremely revealing so be careful because you might be shocked by how many calories you are consuming. With the typical portion sizes at double and even triple what they should be you may be consuming twice to three times what your body needs to maintain its weight. Be cautious of the snacking and the little bites you take here and there. They can add up a lot. This is also a great exercise to educate yourself about how many calories are in items. Start your own journal or use an online calorie counter. To find your recommended caloric intake check out mypyramid.gov. This website can also be extremely useful in showing you were to cut back and what foods to introduce into your diet.

94. Find a Refuge, Restaurant, Spa or Community Center that You Can Get Away from Work and Decompress with the People that Work at the Establishment or with a Friend

Choose a place that is on the way home from work to home but not too close to work.

It would be nice if the place had a walking path close by to take an after work walk before you go home. Expand your community; get to know the people that work there, but do not talk about work.

95. Take 10-Minutes to Relax Your Body and Mind by Doing Deep Breathing and Progressive Muscle Relaxation (PMR) Together

You can do this at your desk or if you an escape to a quiet place that would be better. You cannot be more relaxed after you deep breathe. It is one of the moist efficient ways to reset yourself and calm the inner demons. So go ahead do it, close your eyes and relax, try not to think of anything. Physical tension can lead to mental tension and it does feel good.

PMR is the act of relaxing all your muscles in your body. You first tense up your muscle and then relax it. Start with your hands and more up you arm to your neck and them down your chest, hips and finally all your leg muscles. Don't leave out a muscle. So, if you have a tense moment in your day, do both of these in succession and you will be completely relaxed in your mind and body.

96. Get a Massage

Massage therapy is extremely beneficial for your body and your mind. The benefits include: decreasing heart rate and blood pressure, increasing blood circulation and lymph flow, relaxes your muscles, increases range of motion, increases the endorphin (feel good chemicals), reduces muscles spasms, relieves muscle tension, nourishes skin, and improves posture. Really, do you need any other reason?

Make sure you choose a well-trained masseuse who knows their anatomy. Ask them to tell you about where you carry your stress and what you can do at home to relieve it. Discuss what massage options they provide. These could range from relaxation, deep tissue, hot stone, or Thai. You may also want to treat a friend or significant other to a message. Do a couple's massage and take the time to help each other relax.

Drink lots of water before and after a massage to remove toxins that are released during a massage.

97. Do a Body Check For Cancer

Check your body for signs of skin cancers. Look for any moles that have appeared, grown, or changed in size or color. You need to check your entire body and not just areas that have been exposed to the sun. Consult a dermatologist immediately if you notice anything suspicious. Self-breast and prostate exams should be done monthly. Check for lumps, inconsistencies, or any changes that may have occurred. Lymph nodes Common initial signs of cancer include fatigue and unexplained weight loss. Do not become alarmed, these can be symptoms of other aliments, but do not delay in consulting your doctor.

98. Look at Your Feet Critically

Oh no, the fungus among us. The feet often get neglected. We need to look for feet ulcers, nail and toe fungus, feet swelling. Ulcers can become infected. Generally feet get bacterial or fungal infection. Bacterial feet infections are accompanied by redness, warmth, tenderness and sometimes swelling. Feet swelling can also be a sign of kidney, heart or liver disease. Diabetics lose feeling in their feet and may have terrible ulcers, burns or infections and do not even know it because they cannot feel much pain. If you are a diabetic, you should have your feet examined by the doctor at least every 6 months. Studies have shown that one reason feet problems are forgotten is the shoes remain on and the patient forgets there was a problem down there, out of site out of mind. So remember to take off you shoes to show the doctor if you have feet problem

99. Use Informative Websites to Create a Grocery List Before You Go to the Store

Studies show that people who plan their meals in advance eat healthier and consume less fat and calories.

Useful website include HYPERLINK "http://www.mypyramid.com" www.mypyramid.com or even websites that offer low fat recipes. Take a few minutes before you grocery shop to plan meals and healthy snacks.

Keep a running list on your refrigerator of all the healthy items you enjoy and need to replace. When you go to the grocery store armed with a list you are less likely to be swayed by unhealthy impulse buys. If you have the visual of a list on the frig door you may also reconsider buying unhealthy items.

Now your kitchen will be stocked with healthier choices and you won't feel tempted by the cheese doozzles that jumped into your cart last time.

100. Develop a Home Aerobic Program and Create a Space For It

Do a half hour workout at home in front of the television – make sure the priority is the workout and not the show, so chose the show carefully. If you have a treadmill or stationary bike at home then you are all set. If you don't, then get ideas from workout shows. There are several exercises that can be done in front of the television.

Check you target heart rate during the commercials.

If you simply cannot vigorously workout and watch television, develop a body-stretching program. I know you can stretch and watch television at the same time.

101. Develop and Morning and Evening Teeth Brushing, Flossing, Face and Body Ritual

Brushing your teeth is mandatory, and not just for cosmetics, breath issues, or even just to avoid long visits to the dentist. The health of your mouth is vital to the health of your whole body. It is important to understand that good hygiene of the teeth and gums will prevent you from getting more infections. Having more plaque and gum disease means you have more bacteria that are resident in your mouth. Having more bacteria around in your mouth results in higher likelihood of developing upper and lowers respiratory infections (colds, bronchitis and pneumonia) as well as other infections as the stomach infections or gastritis. So brushing and flossing is more important than just making your teeth look pretty. To keep young, you should always put a face cream on your face at night.

TIPS FOR THE M.D.

The Complete Physical

A complete physical entails a look at the major systems. It starts with the four vital signs and progresses to the different body systems from head to toe. If you have noticed any physical changes, increased leg swelling, change in color or shape of moles since the last time you were examined, point these changes out to your doctor.

102. Take a Confidence Check and Ask Yourself, Do I Feel Good About Myself? Then Do an Affirmation (a positive statement about yourself)

There have been studies for self-esteem and stress. When we have a lower self-esteem, we are less capable of effectively dealing with stress. To feel good about ourselves and to be able to interact effectively we must have confidence. Repeating affirmations to yourself is a powerful way to build confidence. You do this regularly and you subconscious will take over and one day you will not know where that internal confidence came from.

Do a body affirmation, such as "I have a great smile or I look good". Also do a mind affirmation, for example I am a creative person. I can get through this day with a smile. It might feel a little silly at first but affirmations have been shown to elevate your mood. If they do nothing else at least you can laugh for a few moments in the morning.

103. Get the Recommended Amount of Sleep

Sleep is extremely important for your physical and mental health. Sleep deprivation has been linked to the following: impaired glucose tolerance, increased carbohydrate craving, a weakened immune system, increased risk of cancer, decreased alertness and ability to focus, hardening of the arteries, depression and irritability, and it has been linked to obesity. No one wants any of that. Lack of sleep is not only detrimental to our health but prevents us from handling the stresses of our lives.

When you are maximally stressed, you need energy to fight stress, so sleep is paramount.

104. Take a Full Day Off With Your Significant Other and Do Something In the Spur of the Moment

Plan your own spring break with your significant other. Meet in the morning and take a half hour and plan out a mini vacation in the city or town where you live. Pretend you are a tourist and take in those parks, restaurants, trails or sites you always wanted to see.

Both working together to figure out how to have maximal fun will draw you closer together. Don't laugh guys, it works and it is what you make out it. It can be a great adventure.

SPRING TIPS PLANNER

Choose your two tips per week and place them under the heading, below called Tip #.

Put a line through each chosen tip after you have mastered it.

	Date	Tip #
Week 1	_____	_____
Week 2	_____	_____
Week 3	_____	_____
Week 4	_____	_____
Week 5	_____	_____
Week 6	_____	_____
Week 7	_____	_____
Week 8	_____	_____
Week 9	_____	_____
Week 10	_____	_____
Week 11	_____	_____
Week 12	_____	_____
Week 13	_____	_____

FEEL GOOD SPRING TRACKER

Ideal Body Weight and Deviance +/- from the Ideal

Ideal Body Weight _____

March 20 _____
April weight *(within the 1st week)* _____
May weight *(within the 1st week)* _____
June weight *(within the 1st week)* _____

Total Calorie Intake Maintenance, Weight Loss, to Build Muscle
(your goals may change throughout the year, see www.feelgoodhealthnow.com)

Total Daily Calorie/Fat Gram/
    Protein Gram Intake for Maintenance _____
Total Daily Calorie/Fat Gram/
    Protein Gram Intake for Weight Loss _____
Total Daily Calorie/Fat Gram/
    Protein Intake to Build Muscle _____

Target Heart Rate for Aerobic Exercise
(see www.feelgoodhealthnow.com)

Moderate Intensity THR _____
High Intensity THR _____

FEEL GOOD SPRING

Stressors: *(work, family, personal, financial or environmental)*
_____
_____
_____

Plan to cope with above stressors: _____
_____
_____
_____

Average Feel Good Score (1 to 10)
("1" is Completely Lousy and "10" is Blissful)

March 20   _____
April *(within the 1st week)* Date/Score   _____
May *(within the 1st week)* Date/Score   _____
June *(within the 1st week)* Date/Score   _____

Tips or life changes that increased your feel good score:
_____
_____
_____
_____
_____
_____
_____

… FEEL GOOD HEALTH

The Health & Happiness Planner

Body & Mind Inventory Section

Dominic Gaziano, M.D.

HEALTH & HAPPINESS PLANNER

Body and Mind Inventory Section

The sections below are an effort to put in one place the medical, fitness, and weight reminders to keep you on track. We all get busy and forget important health care tasks such as having our teeth cleaned by the dentist every six months. Before we know it three years go by and our teeth and gums are hurting.

This section is designed for you to fill-out and to show to your doctor. Your doctor can easily assess your medical conditions from the following chart. It is also designed to keep you on track with your weight maintenance goals as well as your aerobic exercise goals. Another section is designed to help you identify your stressors and for you to discover ways to cope with them to help you feel better.

Medical History

Primary Care Doctor *(Internist, Family Medicine or Gynecology doctor)*
_____

Medical Conditions_____
_____
_____
_____
_____

HEALTH & HAPPINESS PLANNER

Medications_____
_____
_____
_____
_____

Allergies_____
_____
_____
_____
_____
_____

Yearly physical *(doctor/date)*_____
_____

Surgeries_____
_____
_____
_____

Hospitalizations_____
_____
_____
_____

Cholesterol level_____

Self-Exams and Date Completed_____
_____
_____

Skin survey_____
_____

Breast Self-exam (women) – *(once a month after your period)*____
_____
_____
_____
_____

Testicular Self-exams (men) – *(once a month)*_____
_____
_____
_____
_____

Medical Appointments

Primary Care Doctor
History of Visits (mm/dd/yyyy):
Example: (08/15/2006), (11/12/2007), (02/22/2008)

Date:_____
_____
_____

HEALTH & HAPPINESS PLANNER

Dentist/Dental Hygienist *(at least twice per year)* _____
_____
_____

Optomologist/Optometrist *(recommended once ever two year)* ___
_____
_____

Other Medical appointments_____
_____
_____
_____

Recurring stressors: *(stressors that occur frequently throughout the year)*_____
_____
_____
_____
_____
_____

Plan to cope with recurring stressors: _____
_____
_____
_____
_____
_____
_____

Tips or lifestyle changes that resulted in the highest feel good score for the year _____
_____
_____
_____
_____
_____
_____
_____

Special considerations for High Blood Pressure Patients and Diabetics

If you have high blood pressure, you should consult with your doctor on the frequency of your visits. You may need to visit the doctor more frequently depending on the severity and the degree of control you may have with your blood pressure.

If you are diabetic, you should check your blood sugars four times a day, before each meal and at bedtime. You should have lab work done at least every six months. You should have your eyes and feet checked yearly.

FEEL GOOD
HEALTH
INDEX

Allergic reactions, 19
Anaphylactic reactions, 19
Anxiety, 91,97-98
Aromatherapy, 131
Body Mass Index (BMI), 29,70-71
Calorie count, 124,127
Cancer prevention, 123,139
Carcinogens, 123,135
Cholesterol analysis, 56-57
Contact dermatitis, 21
Dietary portions, 66
Deep breathing, 136
Depression, 90, 94, 97
Dysthymia, 89
Exercise and calorie burn, 94
Exercise ball, 134
Exercise capabilities, 29
Fat grams, 99
Fats (trans, saturated and unsaturated), 99,132-133
Fiber composition and health benefits, 51
Flu shot, 60
Food guide pyramid, 133,134
Foot care, 139
Grocery list, 140

INDEX

Home aerobic program, 141
Ideal body weight, 28,38-39
Influenca, 87
Laughter groups, 132
Lip care, 105
Low back pain, 53
Message, 139
Obesity, 70-71
Omega-3 fatty acids, 106
Overweight, 70-71
Personal trainer selection, 103
Post traumatic stress disorder, 63
Posture, 69
Pulse, 127
Resistance (weight) training, 100
Sleep, 130,143
Stress, 121-122
Stress score, 136
Support system, 136
Target heart rate (THR), 125,134
Upper respiratory infection (URI), 87-89
Workout efficiency, 129
Yearly physical, 59

FEEL GOOD ALL YEAR!

For more Feel Good Health visit
www.feelgoodhealthnow.com

ABOUT THE AUTHOR

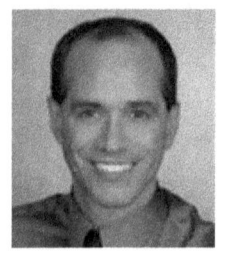

Dominic Gaziano, M.D. is a practicing General Internal Medicine physician in Chicago and BBC World recognized wellness practitioner. He is the director of Body and Mind Medical Wellness Clinic and has made numerous television appearances as a medical expert on health, fitness and nutrition. Dr. Gaziano was appointed to the Chicago Fitness Council, Mayor Daley's health and fitness task force. He served as Medical Director of the Advocate Illinois Masonic Integrative Medicine department for 3 years and now lectures regularly on integrative approaches to anxiety and depression to doctors and other healthcare providers. Dr. Gaziano is also a regular wellness and stress management lecturer to the community.

Having completed his medical research fellowship at Northwestern University in Chicago, Dr Gaziano went on to pursue some of his other passions including writing and television producing. He completed the advanced two-year playwriting workshop at Chicago's Victory Gardens Theater, the 2001 Tony Award-winner for Best Regional Theater. He also graduated the Second City acting and writing comedy school. Dr. Gaziano then went on to recruit Second City talent for his first TV show, Fitness Follies... the Saturday Night Live for fitness. He then created and produced 33 episodes of the internationally syndicated Health and Lifestyles Weekly, a half hour television magazine show that gives tips for healthy living.

Dr. Gaziano comes from a long line of doctors; his father is a practicing pulminologist. Three of his four brothers also have taken the Hippocratic Oath.

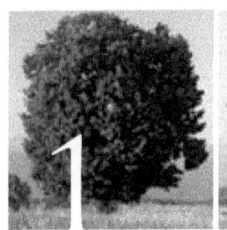
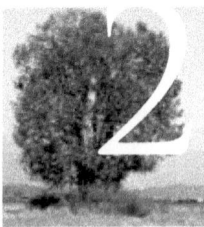
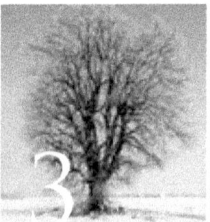
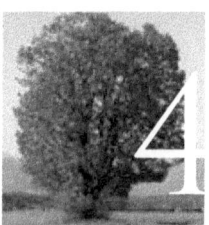